Children, Gender and Families in Mediterranean Welfare States

Children's Well-Being: Indicators and Research Series

Volume 2

This new series focuses on the subject of measurements and indicators of children's well being and their usage, within multiple domains and in diverse cultures. More specifically, the series seeks to present measures and data resources, analysis of data, exploration of theoretical issues, and information about the status of children, as well as the implementation of this information in policy and practice. By doing so it aims to explore how child indicators can be used to improve the development and the well being of children.

With an international perspective the series will provide a unique applied perspective, by bringing in a variety of analytical models, varied perspectives, and a variety of social policy regimes.

Children's Well-Being: Indicators and Research will be unique and exclusive in the field of measures and indicators of children's lives and will be a source of high quality, policy impact and rigorous scientific papers.

For further volumes:
http://www.springer.com/series/8162

Mimi Ajzenstadt · John Gal
Editors

Children, Gender and Families in Mediterranean Welfare States

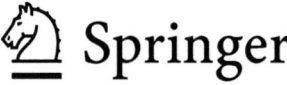 Springer

Editors
Mimi Ajzenstadt
Paul Baerwald School of Social Work &
  Social Welfare
The Institute of Criminology, Faculty of Law
The Hebrew University of Jerusalem
Mount Scopus
91905 Jerusalem
Israel
mimi@mscc.huji.ac.il

John Gal
Paul Baerwald School of Social Work &
  Social Welfare
The Hebrew University of Jerusalem
Mount Scopus
91905 Jerusalem
Israel
msjgsw@mscc.huji.ac.il

ISBN 978-90-481-8841-3   e-ISBN 978-90-481-8842-0
DOI 10.1007/978-90-481-8842-0
Springer Dordrecht Heidelberg London New York

Library of Congress Control Number: 2010925146

Springer is part of Springer Science+Business Media (www.springer.com)

Contents

Contributors

Mimi Ajzenstadt Paul Baerwald School of Social Work & Social Welfare, The Institute of Criminology, Faculty of Law, Hebrew University of Jerusalem, 91905 Jerusalem, Israel, mimi@mscc.huji.ac.il

Valeria Fargion Department of Political Science and Sociology, University of Florence, Florence, Italy, valeria.fargion@unifi.it

John Gal Paul Baerwald School of Social Work & Social Welfare, Hebrew University of Jerusalem, 91905 Jerusalem, Israel, msjgsw@mscc.huji.ac.il

Anat Guy Department of Behavioral Sciences, College of Management Academic Studies, Hebrew University, Rishon LeZion, 75190 Jerusalem, Israel, msgai@mscc.huji.ac.il

Theano Kallinikaki Professor of Social Work, Department of Social Administration, Democritus University of Thrace, Komotini, Greece, thkallin@socadm.duth.gr

Azer Kılıç Max Planck Institute for the Study of Societies, Cologne, Germany, azerkilic@gmail.com

Hadas Mandel Tel-Aviv University, Tel-Aviv, Israel, hadasm@post.tau.ac.il

James R. McDonell Institute on Family and Neighborhood Life, Clemson University, 225 S. Pleasantburg Dr., McAlister Square, Suite B11, Greenville, SC 29607, USA, jmcdnll@clemson.edu

Thomas Olk Martin-Luther-Universität Halle/Wittenberg Institut für Pädagogik, Franckeplatz 1; Haus 6, 06099 Halle/Saale, Germany, thomas.olk@paedagogik.uni-halle.de

Celia Valiente Universidad Carlos III, Madrid, Spain, valiente@polsoc.uc3m.es

Children, Gender, and Families in Mediterranean Welfare States: An Introduction

John Gal and Mimi Ajzenstadt

The closely intertwined concepts of children, gender, and families have moved to the fore in debates and research on the welfare state in recent years. Researchers, policy-makers, and civil society advocacy groups have all participated in discussions on the diverse aspects of social policies relating to children, gender, and families. This is hardly surprising given the growing understanding that policies relating to these social categories have implications for crucial aspects of the welfare state and its impact upon the lives of its citizens. The sustainability of the welfare state and its demography; the structuring of the labor market and economic productivity; gender equality and the division of labor within and outside of the home; the wellbeing (or, as Ben-Arie & George, 2006 and others have suggested, the "wellbecoming"), of children – these are just some of the issues that are directly linked to these policies.

Political, social, and economic transformations, such as privatization and globalization, have impacted governmental and public attitudes towards basic values supporting the welfare state (see for example, Rhodes, 1996) and brought these issues to the forefront of academic and public debate. These have led to the creation of new modes of state interventions (Ajzenstadt & Rosenhek, 2000). The hollowing of the state (Jessop, 1994; Rhodes, 1994) and changes in the governance of nations has led to the creation of new social spaces, where social actors, mainly NGOs, are gradually replacing the state institutions traditionally responsible for protecting individual rights and needs (Katan & Lowenstein, 2009). This development has provided the necessary space to debate and negotiate ideas about issues such as the role of the state and its responsibility towards citizens. Children and women, groups that are usually among the vulnerable and marginalized group, have found themselves in the foci of such policies and debates.

The goal of this volume is to make a modest contribution to these ongoing discussions by focusing upon issues relating to children, gender, and families in welfare states in a geographically defined region – that of the Mediterranean. While there has been some interesting and valuable research on these issues in individual welfare states in this region and occasional comparative studies comprising a number of these nations (Andreotti et al., 2001; Leibfried, 1992; Matsaganis, Ferrera, Capucha, & Moreno, 2003; Ferrera, 1996; MIRE, 1997; Naldini, 2003; Rhodes, 1997), attempts to undertake a more integrated overview of the social policies of the countries in this region have been particularly limited (for an exception to this, see Petmesidou & Papatheodorou, 2006). The underlying assumption in this volume is that despite the diversity of welfare states bordering the Mediterranean Sea, some interesting commonalities are shared by these nations. Indeed, in his contribution to this volume Gal has described these nations as belonging to an extended family of welfare states that share some common characteristics and outcomes, one of which is the role of the family. By bringing together case analyses of the welfare states in the Mediterranean which focus on children, gender, and families, we maintain that it is possible to shed light on aspects of social policy that do not necessarily emerge in most discussions of these issues in the literature.

The rationale inherent in a volume that focuses on a group of welfare states is of course embedded in the welfare regime typology notion that has dominated much of the comparative social policy literature over the last two decades. The publication of Esping Andersen's seminal work, *The Three Worlds of Welfare Capitalism* in 1990 (and his related 1999 book), which distinguished between three welfare regimes, became a landmark for comparative work of social policies in various countries. Esping-Andersen regarded his typology as a useful tool for comparison between welfare states because it allowed "for greater analytical parsimony and help[s] us to see the forest rather than myriad trees" (1999, p. 73). The publication led to a proliferation of works that adopted diverse lines of inquiry.

This approach has generated varied critiques (see the discussion in Wildeboer Schut, Vrooman, & de Beer, 2001). One such critical response to the concept of welfare regimes and its value as an analytical tool for a comparative analysis was that of Kasza (2002). He questioned the validity of efforts to identify a coherent set of policies in one regime or even in one country due to the complexity of processes of policy development and policy implementations. Such processes are dynamic and are shaped by diverse sets of external forces and by the ideas and beliefs of those responsible for the ongoing formulation and implementation of policy.

Other scholars have sought to adopt the notion of welfare regimes, claiming that the various regimes should be perceived as ideal types, which facilitate a useful comparison between the social policies of different welfare states. Nevertheless they have criticized the limited scope of the original typology (see a review of these in Arts & Gelissen, 2002). One major trend in this literature is that which seeks to modify and expand the welfare states included in the typology suggested by Esping-Andersen. In particular, scholars have sought to identify distinguishing characteristics in the organization of social policies in various countries, assessing whether they can be classified according to Esping-Andersen's welfare types, or if they can be seen as forming a distinct regime.

Thus, various authors have suggested adding additional welfare regime types, that encompass Southern European nations (Bonoli, 1997; Ferrera, 1996), an "East Asian" or "Confucian" welfare regime (Jones, 1993; Kwon, 1997), and a "Radical" or "Antipodean" welfare regime type, which distinguishes Australia and New Zealand from other liberal regimes (Castles & Mitchell, 1991). A more recent debate has emerged concerning the possibility of including transition nations within the original model (see, for example, Fenger, 2007).

Another line of inquiry is aimed at providing empirical data in relation to various policies adopted by countries in the different regimes; measuring, in particular, their outcomes. These studies utilize a variety of indicators and advanced research methods in order to examine the persistence of significant distinctions in social policy organizations which can be classified into identifiable welfare regimes (see for example, Saint-Arnaud & Bernard, 2003).

A group of studies has attempted to examine the regime analytical framework by highlighting a specific policy. These works limit the comparative investigation to a detailed examination of a specific domain or a cluster of social policies across welfare regimes. Gallie and Paugam (2000) for example, offered a comprehensive unemployment-centered framework locating the employment and unemployment policies in various welfare regimes. Similarly, Matznetter (2002) focused on social housing policy and its relations to the various welfare regimes. Such an approach enables a more detailed analysis of the various dimensions of such a policy within a comparative examination.

Adopting a similar focused approach, feminist scholars have argued that welfare state literature in general, and welfare regime studies in particular, have ignored the gender dimension of the welfare state (see for example Hobson, 1994; Lewis & Ostner, 1995; Sainsbury, 1994, 1999). Challenging this gender omission, they suggested a new welfare state typology which would include policies related to women's experience in the welfare state, adding, for example, such variables as unpaid work to labor-related work to the welfare state analytical framework. They sought to examine welfare regimes by comparing institutional and political arrangements and their impact on women's status and social role in the welfare state (Orloff, 1993; O'Connor, 1996). In addition, they have called for a more nuanced analysis that takes into account the effect of ethnicity and class when examining the different experiences of women (Williams, 1995). Others (Bambra, 2004), however claimed that the original regime typology is not gender blind and when issues such as decommodification or defamilization are brought to the forefront of the regime framework, women's experiences of the welfare state can be compared across the different regimes.

A final line of inquiry stemming from Esping-Anderson's work locates welfare regimes within a nexus of comparative attitude research (see for example Bean & Papadakis, 1998; Jæger, 2006; Svallfors, 2003). These works claim that attitudes towards social policies play an important role in policy formation and implementation, and thus, a comparison of attitudes across various models adds to our understanding of the dynamic of the welfare regime discourse.

The chapters in this volume touch upon many of the themes raised in a comparative approach to the study of social policy and the welfare state. The book is divided to four parts. The initial part of the volume introduces key theoretical concepts related to comparative research and its relevance to the welfare states in the Mediterranean regime. Thus, Olk employs a comparison between welfare states in order to better understand policies towards children. In her chapter, Mandel focuses upon issues of gender and economic inequality in welfare states. McDonell then moves the discussion to the realm of families, employing a US case study.

The second part sets the scene by focusing more specifically upon the Mediterranean region. In his article Gal seeks to make the case for regarding the welfare states in the Mediterranean region as an extended family of nations, by discussing three themes common to all Mediterranean welfare states – religion, family, and clientelism.

Country studies of Mediterranean welfare states comprise a third part of this volume. In the chapters in this part Fargion (Italy), Valiente (Spain), Ajzenstadt (Israel), Kiliç (Turkey), and Kallinikaki (Greece) seek to examine social policy developed in these Mediterranean countries. While not attempting to classify social policies in this area within a specific regime, the chapters do identify similar patterns related to social policies in these states. Most of the studies employ a historical narrative methodology, tracing the processes leading to the development of policies by contextualizing them within the wider social, economic, and cultural context. They underscore the role of internal and external forces in shaping policies and the way they are implemented. This historicity allows the authors to compare various arrangements for welfare provision at local, national, and international levels.

The fourth and final part of the volume contains a cross-national comparison of Mediterranean welfare states. Here, Guy offers quantitative data that underscores the similarities and differences between these nations and between groupings of them.

The chapters in this book focus on social policies targeting children, women, and families. This wide angle offers a useful perspective on social policies by analyzing policies related to childcare and welfare, unpaid work and provision of care to those who are not able to care for themselves, as part of one institutional arrangement spread across various policy arenas. The chapters highlight how key social concepts such as the nature of citizenship, the role of women and the family, the nature of childhood, the role of religious beliefs, and the public/private dichotomy shape the provision and the use of welfare services in the interrelated social policies of the combined arena. This focus allows us to identify commonalities and differences between the various states in relation to the policy arena targeting women, children, and families. Hopefully, the chapters provide a useful framework for further thought, theory, and research at the policy, discursive, and institutional levels, and identify patterns of convergence and sites of overlap that deserve further analysis.

This book idea originated at an international workshop organized by the Social Policy Research Group of the Paul Baerwald School of Social Work and Social Welfare held at the Hebrew University of Jerusalem in June 2008. The conference was devoted to the theme of Gender, Children, and Families in Mediterranean Welfare States. The presentations and discussions in the conference inspired us to continue this line of inquiry, in an attempt to extend the relevant theoretical and empirical issues. The conference was sponsored by the Authority of Research and Development, the Federmann School of Public Policy and Government, the Lafer Center for Women and Gender Studies, the Levi Eshkol Institute for Social Economic and Political Research in Israel, the Cherrick Center for the Study of Zionism, the Yishuv and the State of Israel, the Minerva Centers for Human Rights at the Hebrew University of Jerusalem and Tel-Aviv University, the Italian Embassy in Israel, and the JDC Tevet Organization.

Our appreciation is due to the various participants in the workshop who provided us with valuable insights and ideas. These included Dr. Asher Ben-Arie, Prof. Abraham Doron, Dr. Michal Frenkel, Prof. David Levi Faur, Michal Koreh, Ronen Mandelkern, Prof. Michael Shalev, Prof. Peter Taylor-Gooby, Prof. Uri Yanay, and Prof. Joseph Zeira. In addition, we would like to thank Roni Holler who has helped us throughout the process and to Mara Getz Sheftel for her editorial work. Finally, we are very grateful to the editorial staff at Springer and the book series editor, Dr. Asher Ben-Arie, for facilitating the publication of this volume.

References

Ajzenstadt, M., & Rosenhek, Z. (2000). Privatization and new modes of state intervention: The long-term care program in Israel. *Journal of Social Policy, 29*, 247–262.

Andreotti, A., Garcia, S. M., Gomez, A., Hespanha, P., Kazepov, Y., & Mingione, E. (2001). Does a Southern European model exist? *Journal of European Area Studies, 9*(1), 43–62.

Arts, W., & Gelissen, J. (2002). Three worlds of welfare capitalism or more? A state-of-the-art report. *Journal of European Social Policy, 12*(2), 137–158.

Bambra, C. (2004). The worlds of welfare: Illusory and gender blind? *Social Policy and Society, 3*(3), 201–211.

Bean, C., & Papadakis, E. (1998). A comparison of mass attitudes towards the welfare state in different institutional regimes, 1985–1990. *International Journal of Public Opinion Research, 10*(3), 211–236.

Ben-Arie, A., & Goerge, R. (2006). Measuring and monitoring children's well-being: The policy process. In A. Ben-Arie & R. Goerge (Eds.), *Indicators of children's well-being: Understanding their role, usage, and policy influence* (pp. 21–30). Dordrecht, Netherlands: Springer.

Bonoli, G. (1997). Classifying welfare states: A two dimensional approach. *Journal of Social Policy, 26*(3), 351–372.

Castles, F. G., & Mitchell, D. (1991). *Three worlds of welfare capitalism or four?* Canberra: Australian National University, Graduate Program in Public Policy.

Ferrera, M. (1996). The "Southern" model of welfare in Social Europe. *Journal of European Social Policy, 6*(1), 17–37.

Fenger, H. J. M. (2007). Welfare regimes in Central and Eastern Europe: Incorporating post-communist countries in a welfare regime typology. *Contemporary Issues and Ideas in Social Sciences, 3*(2), 1–30.

Esping-Anderson, G. (1990). *The three worlds of welfare capitalism*. Princeton, NJ: Princeton University Press.

Esping-Andersen, G. (1999). *Social foundations of post-industrial economies*. Oxford: Oxford University Press.

Gallie, D. & Paugam, S. (Eds.). (2000). *Welfare regimes and the experience of unemployment in Europe*. Oxford: Oxford University Press.

Hobson, B. (1994). Solo mothers, social policy regimes, and the logics of gender. In D. Sainsbury (Ed.), *Gendering welfare states* (pp. 170–187). London: Sage.

Jæger, M. M. (2006). Welfare regimes and attitudes towards redistribution: The regime hypothesis revisited. *European Sociological Review, 22*(2), 157–170.

Jessop, B. (1994). Post-Fordism and the state. In A. Amin (Ed.), *Post-Fordism: A reader* (pp. 251–279). Oxford: Blackwell.

Jones, C. (1993). The pacific challenge. In C. Jones (Ed.), *New perspectives on the welfare state in Europe* (pp. 184–203). London: Routledge.

Katan, J., & Lowenstein, A. (2009). Privatization trends in welfare services and their impact upon Israel as a welfare state. In J. Hendricks & J. Powell (Eds.), *The welfare state in post-industrial society* (pp. 311–332). New York: Springer.

Kasza, G. J. (2002). The illusion of welfare 'regimes'. *Journal of Social Policy, 31*, 271–287.

Kwon, H. J. (1997). Beyond European welfare regimes: comparative perspectives on East Asian welfare systems. *Journal of Social Policy, 26*(4), 467–484.

Leibfried, S. (1992). Towards a European welfare state? On integrating poverty regimes into the European Community. In Z. Ferge & J. E. Kolberg (Eds.), *Social policy in a changing Europe* (pp. 245–280). Frankfurt: Campus Verlag.

Matsaganis, M., Ferrera, M., Capucha, L., & Moreno, L. (2003). Mending nets in the South: Anti-poverty policies in Greece, Italy, Portugal and Spain. *Social Policy and Administration, 37*(1), 639–655.

Matznetter, W. (2002). Social housing policy in a conservative welfare state: Austria as an example. *Urban Studies, 39*(2), 265–282.

MIRE. (1997). *Comparing social welfare systems in Southern Europe: Vol. 3 Florence conference.* Paris: MIRE.

Lewis, J., & Ostner, I. (1995). Gender and the evolution of European social policy. In S. Leibfreid & P. Pierson (Eds.), *European social policy: Between fragmentation and integration* (pp. 159–193). Washington, DC: Brookings Institute.

Naldini, M. (2003). *The family in the Mediterranean welfare states.* London: Frank Cass.

O'Connor, J. S. (1996). Gendering welfare state regimes. *Current Sociology, 44*(2), 1–130.

Orloff, A. (1993). Gender and the social rights of citizenship: The comparative analysis of gender relations and welfare states. *American Sociological Review, 58*, 303–328.

Petmesidou, M., & Papatheodorou, C. (Eds.). (2006). *Poverty and social deprivation in the Mediterranean.* London: Zed.

Rhodes, R. A. W. (1994). The hollowing out of the state: The changing nature of the public service in Britain. *Political Quarterly Review, 65*, 137–151.

Rhodes, M. (1996). Globalization and West European welfare states: A critical review of recent debates. *Journal of European Social Policy, 6*(4), 305–327

Rhodes, M. (Ed.). (1997). *Southern European welfare states: Between crisis and reform.* London: Frank Cass & Co. Ltd.

Saint-Arnaud, S., & Bernard, P. (2003). Convergence or resilience? A hierarchical cluster analysis of the welfare regimes in advanced countries. *Current Sociology, 51*(5), 499–527.

Sainsbury, D. (1999). Gender, policy regimes and politics. In D. Sainsbury (Ed.), *Gender and welfare state regimes* (pp. 245–293). Oxford: Oxford University Press.

Sainsbury, D. (Ed.). (1994). *Gendering welfare states.* London: Sage.

Svallfors, S. (2003). Welfare regimes and welfare options: A comparison of eight western countries. *Social Indicators Research, 64*, 495–520.

Wildeboer Schut, J. M., Vrooman, J. C., & de Beer, P. (2001). *On worlds of welfare. Institutions and their effects in eleven welfare states.* The Hague: Social and Cultural Planning Office the Netherlands.

Williams, F. (1995). Race/ethnicity, gender, and class in welfare states: A framework for comparative analysis. *Social Politics*, Spring, 127–159.

Part I
Key Concepts

Investing in Children? Changes in Policies Concerning Children and Families in European Countries

Thomas Olk

Introduction

Until recently children and families only played a marginal role in welfare politics. Prior to this shift within the political sphere, the main focus was placed upon
protecting (male) workers against the risks associated with industrial work: old age,
sickness, occupational accidents and unemployment. Women and children were protected indirectly by provision offered to the male breadwinner. Choices involving
the structure of the family and the rearing of children were considered private matters. As a consequence, in the developed welfare states, the lion's share of social
spending was dedicated to pensions and health, while the share of the social budget
that was spent on children and families only represented a marginal sum.

In this respect a profound shift has taken place within the last 10–15 years.
Children and families now play a more important role within the developed welfare
states. For instance, some countries (i.e. Canada and UK) launched ambitious and
comprehensive political programs to fight child poverty. In many countries there
are currently initiatives to improve the conditions for families with children – the
majority of which aim at improving the reconciliation of family and work, introducing family friendly working hours, and the expansion of spots in childcare centres.
Furthermore, due to increased expectations of the economy in regard to the skill
level of workers, many countries have focused on a reform of the educational system and a modernisation of the system of early childcare and education. While
this trend began as early as the 1980s, it is only within the last decade that it has
gained significant momentum. Accordingly, an analysis of social spending in 21
industrialised countries carried out by Gabel and Kamerman (cf. 2006) comes to the
conclusion that despite some country variations spending on children and families
has increased in most countries between 1980 and 2001. This holds true regardless

T. Olk (✉)
Martin-Luther-Universität Halle/Wittenberg Institut für Pädagogik, Franckeplatz 1; Haus 6, 06099
Halle/Saale, Germany
e-mail: thomas.olk@paedagogik.uni-halle.de

M. Ajzenstadt, J. Gal (eds.), *Children, Gender and Families in Mediterranean
Welfare States*, Children's Well-Being: Indicators and Research 2,
DOI 10.1007/978-90-481-8842-0_1, © Springer Science+Business Media B.V. 2010

of the kind of measure: spending as a percentage of GDP, spending as a percentage of social protections expenditures, or spending per child.

Additionally, international organisations have been contributing to this trend. For example, the OECD (cf. 2001, 2006) propagated the development of early childhood education and care (ECEC) as an important contribution to a successful transition into the knowledge society. According to the Lisbon Strategy, the EU announced new goals for policies concerning children and families as well as introduced benchmarks for evaluating the implementation of these goals in the member states. Finally, in an influential evaluation completed for the EU Presidency, Esping-Andersen and his colleagues argued for a concept of a "child-centred social investment strategy" (cf. 2002).

This shift in the political priorities of the developed welfare states is usually explained in terms of changing economic, social, and political conditions. According to this line of thinking new challenges like the aging of populations, falling fertility rates, and changing structure of families not to mention the coming of the knowledge-based society automatically cause the development of a new political strategy concerning children and families. If this view were correct, then all countries would have to react more or less in the same manner to the global challenges. However, as recent history has shown this is not the case. Confronted with the same challenges some countries develop new political programmes and priorities whereas others do not. Furthermore, the analysis of the OECD Social Expenditure database (SOCX) comes to the conclusion, that there are changing family policy goals focusing on such things as reconciling work and family responsibilities, providing incentives to work, and enhancing the development of young children by means of early childhood care and education programmes. However, there is a substantial variation in the commitment to these new goals by the countries studied. This provokes the question as to "why some countries have placed children higher on their political agenda than others, and why some countries have managed to increase or sustain more generous policies while others have not" (Gabel & Kamerman, 2006, p. 161).

The Role of Ideas in the Field of Child and Family Policies

To sum up: it is not enough to explain policy change by referring to external pressures and problems as well as to national policy legacies and institutional arrangements. Accordingly, the recent literature on policy change stresses the importance of social-learning, ideas, and discourses for political analysis and explaining policy change (cf. Yee, 1996; Hall, 1993; Schmidt, 2002; Schmidt & Radaelli, 2004; see Kuebler, 2007 for an analysis of family policies). It is assumed that under specific conditions ideas and discourses are better able to explain political change than other approaches. This is the case when networks consisting of societal and state actors, confronted with new challenges, are successful in establishing a new definition of political problems and are able to link these new perceptions to new political goals and innovative instruments. The ideational approach does not claim to explain all forms of political change. Occasionally, processes of social learning, ideas, and discourses are the decisive factors in explaining political change. However, discourses can serve to bridge the gap between institutionalist and actor-centred analysis – and thus between structure and agency. Political change cannot be explained merely by referring to reactions of policy-makers to socio-economic trends like the demographic challenge, the process of globalisation or the coming of the knowledge-based society. Depending upon which discourses and political ideas are employed, decision-makers make sense of the given external pressures and problems which they need to identify, as well as link these needs to political strategies and instruments.

Against this backdrop the issue has to be raised as to which discourses and political ideas decision-makers utilise in order to legitimate a major shift in the aims and instruments in the field of children and family policies. In this respect, two approaches are potential candidates: the children's rights approach and the social investment approach. The children's rights approach identifies children as bearers of (social) rights and as fully fledged citizens. In particular, the ratification of the UN Convention on the Rights of the Child in 1989 represents a turning point in the national and international discourses concerning children's rights. Since then, political initiatives to enhance children's rights have been gaining in influence. Following Therborn (cf. 1993), the UN Convention acted as a catalyst in the development of child politics as a separate policy field in many industrialised countries in which the main actors in this policy field are international non-governmental organisations. In the field of social policy, debates on appropriate ways of acknowledging the individual rights and entitlements of children as well as accommodating the process of social policy making to the interests and views of children are gaining ground. Since then, it has been an open and contested issue how and to what extent the citizenship and social rights of children have to be considered within national welfare state regimes.

Whereas the children's rights approach focuses on rights, the social investment approach focuses on the economic value of children. To adapt the advanced western welfare states to changing economic and social conditions the concept of "investing in children" is propagated (cf. Esping-Andersen, 2002, 2005; see Jenson & Saint-Martin, 2003; Lister, 2004, 2006; Dobrowolsky & Jenson, 2005 for a critical analysis of this topic). The idea here is to replace the traditional welfare state by a social investment state, i.e. instead of providing direct economic maintenance the state should invest in human capital. As one of the leading proponents of this view Gøsta Esping-Andersen argues for the concept of a "child-centred social investment strategy" (cf. 2002 see also 2008). Under the conditions of a globalised competitive economy and low birth rates modern states cannot afford for certain population groups to fail to cope with the requirements of the knowledge-based economy. According to this view, the potential advantage of the EU-countries is the result of their stock of human capital; this has to be mobilised to afford the economic growth and welfare of the population. However, the life chances of people are determined to a great extent by influences experienced in their early childhood (cf. Esping-Andersen, 2008). Consequently, the preconditions for school achievement and successful occupational careers must also be improved in early childhood. Therefore, investments in early childhood produce individual returns later on by increasing incomes in the future as well as yielding a social dividend; for the greying population is dependent upon the higher productivity of the next generations of workers.

In the following analysis it is assumed that there is a certain correspondence between the predominant political paradigm, on the one hand, and a specific discourse on the role of children in society, on the other. Between these two factors there is a close interaction: a certain kind of social and political practice of treating children and families is legitimised by specific social constructions of children and childhood. A new political paradigm in the field of policies concerning children and families can only be established by implementing new ideas and values concerning the role and status of childhood and children in the society. Of course, to explain the changes and continuities in childhood over time and within a given society, we need to include a wide variety of factors and processes. These include social, political and economic processes that Allison and Adrian James describe as "the cultural politics of childhood" (cf. 2004). The analysis of the "cultural politics of childhood" must be engaged in the identification of processes "by which these cultural determinants and discourses are put into practice at any given time, in any given culture, to construct 'childhood' in society" (James & James, 2004, p. 7). According to this, Allison and Adrian James identify law as a "key mechanism" for this process of construction and reconstruction of childhood within a given society. As far as the influence of political strategies in a narrower sense – i.e. political programs, measures, and discourses – are focused on analysis, they speak of a "politics of childhood" (cf. 2004 and 2005). This article assumes that in some advanced welfare states we are witnessing a process by which an existing "old" political paradigm in the field of policies concerning children and families is being replaced by a "new" political paradigm. Each political paradigm is associated with a specific social construction of childhood and children. Whereas the "old" political paradigm – based on family responsibility – made parents exclusively responsible for the well-being of their children, the "new" political paradigm interprets children as a human asset, where the responsibility for investing in children is divided between the parents and the state (cf. Jenson, 2004).

If, and to what extent, this new political paradigm of "investing in children" will be implemented in different countries depends on a multitude of factors (cf. Olk & Wintersberger, 2007; see also Qvortrup 2008). It is clear, however, that factors like institutional arrangements and policy legacies or interests still play an important role. Nonetheless, the following analysis demonstrates that in many cases it is primarily the propagation of a new discourse regarding the role and status of children and parents in society that is responsible for the radical changes witnessed in several countries. Hence, it is above all the processes of social learning and discourse policies which can best explain a radical change in policies concerning children and families in some countries. In order to examine this approach, in the rest of the essay I will analyse the children and family policies in Germany, Norway, and Italy with respect to the causes and processes of political change.

The selection of these countries is legitimate for two reasons: Firstly, the potential influence of the type of welfare regime on processes of political learning can be controlled. According to Esping-Andersen's typology (cf. 1990), Germany can be assigned to the conservative welfare regime model, Norway to the social democratic model, and Italy to the Mediterranean welfare model. Secondly, the dynamics of politics concerning children and families are different enough to demonstrate the importance of different factors causing policy change in these countries.

Germany: "Sustainable Family Policy" – Reframing Policies Concerning Children and Families

Until 2002 – the beginning of the second term of the red-green coalition under Chancellor Gerhard Schröder – no one would have guessed that a new paradigm regarding family policy, causing a radical change in political strategies and instruments, would have been possible in Germany. When the Minister of Family Affairs Renate Schmidt took office a new concept under the title "sustainable family policy" was developed and implemented. This was the result of the huge discrepancy perceived between relatively high spending levels for programs and measures related to children and families, on the one hand, and their relatively small impact, on the other. Although Germany ranks relatively high among European nations in terms of spending for families and children– with only Luxembourg providing a more generous child benefit package – the following deficits were found:

- The fertility rate in Germany was 1.35; a rate placing it in the lowest third in international rankings;
- German pupils ranked very low in international school achievement tests (PISA-test);
- Child poverty rates have been on the rise since the late 1980s;
- As compared to other nations, the rate of women's participation (especially mothers) in the labour market was relatively low.

To overcome the deficits of the old family policy a radical policy change was introduced. The new concept of "sustainable family policy" was implemented with the following objectives:

- Fertility rate: to secure the demographic continuance an average fertility rate of 1.7 children per woman needs to be reached;
- Reconciliation of work and family: to increase the participation of women in the labour market as well as the implementation of measures aimed at increasing the fertility rate by means of a better reconciliation of work and family responsibilities;

- Fighting child poverty: instead of focusing on social spending in order to eradicate child and family poverty, an emphasis was placed on increasing the labour market participation of both parents;
- Investing in education: investments in education, especially aimed at expanding slots in early childhood education and care facilities and by expanding the number of all-day schools, are to be made in order to improve the conditions for future economic growth and to prevent child and family poverty.

In order to overcome the marginal status of family policy compared to other fields of policy as well as to make the new concept of family policy more convincing, the new paradigm of "sustainable family policy" was intentionally conceptualised as part of a strategy of economic modernisation. For this reason it was interpreted as a strategy of "economisation of the family policy discourse" (Leitner, 2008). The head of the department for family policy at the Ministry of Family Affairs, Malte Ristau, argues in an article from June 2005 that the Minister of Family Affairs, with the help of the new concept of "sustainable family policy", relies on "the economic charm of the family" (cf. Ristau, 2005, p. 19). In addition, the federal government's stand on the 7th Family Report in 2006 views this change of paradigms in the field of family policy as legitimised by economic arguments: "Families ensure the social growth as well as economic prosperity of our society. Germany cannot afford to waste important potentials for further growth and innovation" (BMFSFJ, 2006, p. XXIV).

Furthermore, the specific objectives of the concept of sustainable family policy must prove their economic viability. For example, increasing the birth rate addresses the labour shortage due to demographic change; an improvement of the system of early childcare and education contributes to the qualification of the future workforce as well as financially relieving the welfare state.

To increase the persuasiveness of the new concept and to gain allies within civil society, scientific experts were employed to communicate the new ideas. Two experts were particularly significant. First, the economist Bert Rürup, advising the German government regarding economic issues, analysed the demographic challenge. He concluded that a stabilisation of the labour supply as a consequence of demographic trends could be reached just by increasing the birth rate and the labour market participation of women. From an economic perspective he argues for a reduction of opportunity costs, especially for educated women (cf. Rürup & Gruesco, 2003).

The sociologist Hans Bertram – simultaneously head of the independent expert commission of the 7th Family Report – stressed in his conclusion the existence of different family and work orientations of women. He argued the importance of taking into account different biographical orientations of women by structuring policies concerning children and families to allow as many women as possible to have children regardless of their orientation toward work and career. In accordance with this line of thinking he advocates an intelligent mix of time politics, infrastructure, and financial transfers (cf. Bertram, Rösler & Ehlert, 2005).

The strategic economisation of the family policy discourse becomes evident when one considers that within the context of the new paradigm each family policy measure will be legitimised by verifying its economic efficiency. The central message is: sustainable family policy pays off![1]

The joint statement of these studies is that the new concept of sustainable family policy is in the genuine interest of enterprises, improves conditions for economic growth, and thus, families represent a good investment! To enforce a real policy change the Minister of Family Affairs needed allies both in the state departments and civil society because, traditionally speaking, family policy in Germany is a weak policy field. The Ministry of Family Affairs is not fully responsible for all measures and programs related to children and families. For example, the Ministry for Financial Affairs is responsible for child benefits and family-oriented taxations. Complicating matters, the federal structure of the German state must also be considered in this equation. This means that the responsibility for family policy is dispersed between all three levels: federal, state and local authorities. This fact alone makes it very difficult to develop a consistent family policy concept. Whereas the federal states (Bundesländer) are responsible for education, the local authorities are responsible for social services for families, children and youths. Furthermore, as a consequence of a recent reform of the federalism the responsibilities of the state, especially in the field of education, have been further weakened. As already mentioned the federal Ministry of Family Affairs, Senior Citizens, Women and Youth (BMFSFJ) is, traditionally speaking, a weak ministry with limited competencies and a small budget. Family Affairs ministers do not have high priority in the Cabinet and their power depends on their relationship with the Chancellor and their popularity with the public. To improve its own power and its ability to persuade other powerful actors the federal Ministry of Family Affairs forged an alliance with influential societal actors prominent in the public realm; individuals from the economic sphere, unions, charities, churches and sciences. The "Alliance for Families" served as a platform for joint activities (Mohn & von der Leyen, 2007).

These influential personalities have helped expand early childcare and education, introduce family-friendly work schedules in businesses, and create and implement a sustainable family policy. The "Local Alliances for Families" was initiated by the Ministry of Family Affairs as a counterpart to the "National Alliance for Families" at the local level. The aim was to encourage local authorities, businesses and non-profit organisations to implement measures to improve the situation of families within a given community. At present, there are 445 "Local Alliances for Families" in

---

[1] In the meantime a number of studies calculating the economic benefit of family policy measures were commissioned by the Ministry of Family Affairs (BMFSFJ). For example, one analysis by the German Institute for Economic Research (DIW) calculates the positive economic effects of the extension of facilities for early childcare and education at all levels of the federal state (central government, federal states and local authorities). Furthermore, in another study, Prognos-AG calculated the economic effects of family friendly measures for small- and midrange businesses. All these studies are available on the Ministry for Family Affairs homepage (www.bmfsfj.de).

Germany. Allies in this movement are local businesses and the regional Chambers of Trade and Commerce.

All in all, with the help of the concept of sustainable family policy the Ministry of Family Affairs managed to implement a new paradigm of policy concerning children and families, to identify new target groups with new social needs and to involve new political actors. For example, by highlighting the issue of reconciliation of family and work responsibilities, the needs of working mothers and caring fathers, and the needs of young children (especially those under the age of three) have become a focal point. Furthermore, additional resources for a sustainable family policy were mobilised by activating new social actors like businesses, business associations, unions, churches, charity organisations and chambers of trade and commerce. Such measures are most important in the context of the new social policy for children and families: increasing the number of slots in early childcare and education for children under the age of three and the new parental leave scheme.[2]

First, the legislation concerning the expansion of early childcare for children under the age of three (Tagesbetreuungsausbaugesetz) was launched in January of 2005. With the help of this law roughly 230,000 additional slots for children under three are to be created by 2010 – closing in on the international standard. Provision rates in Germany had fallen far behind the other European nations – especially compared to the Nordic countries. In 1998 the provision rate in Western Germany was 2.8% and about 36.3% in Eastern Germany; a total of 7% (cf. Jurczyk, Olk, & Zeiher, 2004; Rauschenbach, 2006; Spieß, Berger, & Groh-Samberg, 2008). In accordance with this law, local authorities who are responsible for financing early childcare and education are requested to identify the need for childcare at the local level and to offer no fewer than the number of slots for children of this age whose parents are: both gainfully employed, single parents, participating in vocational courses or in integration measures organised by the new social assistance for the long-term unemployed (Hartz IV). To implement this law 1.5 Billion Euro a year will have been invested through to 2010 (BMFSFJ, 2006, p. 4).

In addition to the reform of the system of early childcare and education for children under 3 years of age, Minister Schmidt aimed at reforming the parental leave scheme during her term. The previous parental leave scheme offered only a very small flat rate compared to wages and incomes (300€) with the consequence that the opportunity costs for the parent who interrupts his/her gainful employment to care for his/her child were very high. In practice it was primarily mothers (more than 90%) who took the existing parental leave scheme. Thus, the central aim of the new parental leave scheme is to reduce the opportunity costs associated with raising

---

[2]In addition to these new measures in the field of family policy, in Spring 2002 the "Future, Education and Care" – 2003–2007 – (IZBB) initiative was launched by the federal government. As a reaction to the results of the PISA-study and the deficits in the supply of afterschool care, the federal government developed the aim to increase the number of all-day schools. 4 Billion Euro was spent by the federal government to enable the Länder to make about 40,000 schools in Germany all-day schools by 2007.

a child – especially for highly educated women. As such, according to this reform, mothers or fathers who interrupt their employment to care for their child receive 67% of their former wages for up to 12 months. To motivate fathers to take more responsibility in caring for their children, initially 3 months of paid parental leave were reserved for the father.

Because of the early federal elections (which took place in 2005 instead of 2006) it was not possible to launch the new parental leave scheme during the red-green coalition's second term. However, the newly formed CDU/CSU and SPD coalition took up the former coalition's initiative and the new Minister of Family Affairs, Ursula von der Leyen (CDU), continued with the family policy of her predecessor Renate Schmidt (SPD). Thus, the German Bundestag adopted the law concerning the new parental leave in September of 2006, and it came into effect in January of 2007. The amount of the new parental leave is 67% of the average net income of the person who cares for the child, up to a maximum of 1,800€ per month. Parents who did not work in the previous months before giving birth are eligible to receive a monthly payment of 300€. The parental leave can even be divided between both parents. However, 2 months are reserved for the parent who continued working, which is usually the father (the so-called "daddy quota"). Lone parents are eligible for a parental leave of up to 14 months. There are several aims involved in the new parental leave policy: The primary aim is to reduce opportunity costs for the caring parent. Furthermore, by reducing the duration of the new parental leave to a maximum of 12 months per person mothers are expected to be better integrated into the labour market. Furthermore, this policy should provide incentives for giving birth to more children. With this reform, it was accepted that families with higher incomes profit more from this law than poorer people, who actually have fewer benefits than under the previous system (they receive 300€ per month, but only for 14 months instead of 24 months).

Conflict between different interest groups has emerged in relation to the "daddy quota" and there was an intensive public debate on this issue. Some members of the CDU/CSU protested against the introduction of the daddy months arguing that the state should not intervene in the private sphere of the family. However, contrary to previous conflicts there was no party cleavage, only a conflict within the CDU/CSU. Because the CDU (a Bavarian regional party) holds a veto in the German Bundesrat (the Chamber of the Federal States) a political compromise was negotiated. Given the strong political consensus across all political parties and given the wide acceptance of the new parental leave scheme by the public, the opponents were not able to prevent the passing of the new law.

After having implemented the new parental leave, the Minister of Family Affairs started a new initiative to expand early childcare, especially for children under 3 years. The new legislation aimed at supporting children (Kinderförderungsgesetz), which became effective as of January 2009, will increase the provision rate for children under 3 years of age from the present 14 to 35% by 2013. Thus, around 500,000 new slots in crèches and with child minders must be created. The federal government will contribute a share of 4 Billion Euro to the total cost of this initiative – 12 Billion Euro (cf. BMFSFJ, 2008).

All in all, with the help of the new concept of "sustainable family policy" the ministry was able to enforce a new social construction of childhood and to establish a new type of parental responsibility. The new policy for children and families is oriented toward the adult-worker family model. Fathers *and* mothers should be engaged in gainful employment to prevent families from falling into poverty, to stabilise the supply of labour in a situation of demographic aging, and finally, to strengthen the economic security of women. Children are no longer rendered as dependent members of their family, but as a "public good" and as an object of investment in human capital. At the same time, we are witnessing a far-reaching reconstruction of childhood. As a consequence of the expansion of early childcare for children under 3 years of age, the construction of a "learning childhood", even in the very early stages of life, is being implemented.

However, so far there is a strong discrepancy between ambitious political goals on the one hand and the real situation on the other. Nearly no effects of the sustainable family policy can be measured. For example, despite the new parental leave the expected increase in births did not take place. According to preliminary estimations, in 2008 approximately 675,000 children were born – ca. 8,000 or 1.1% less than 2007. Only in Eastern Germany was there a slight increase in the fertility rate. According to experts this trend is caused by the new parental leave (cf. Amann, 2006). Furthermore, for the time being the increase in the number of slots in publicly subsidised daycare is nothing but a political aim. Given the monetary restrictions at the local level and the dispersed responsibilities at different federal levels it is not guaranteed that it will be able to create 500,000 new slots within 4 years.

Norway: A Dualistic Model of Policies Concerning Children and Families

Policies concerning children and families in Norway are shaped by the specific "cultural construction of Norden" (cf. Sørensen & Stråth, 1997) as well as by the ideas and values concerning the status and role of children and families in Norwegian society. These are a central part of the Norwegian social model and a specific version of the social democratic welfare regime (cf. Esping-Andersen, 1990). Furthermore, the "Nordic protestant ethic", the specific geography of the country, and the dominance of the traditional industries like fishing, agriculture, forestry and shipping continue to exert a strong influence. Thus, it is no surprise that such principles as independence, autonomy, individuality and personal freedom still play an important role within society and culture. Traditionally speaking, children were and are considered citizens with their own needs, interests and rights, and childhood was accepted as a stage of life with its own inherent value (cf. Satka and Eydal, 2004; Nilsen, 2008).

Thus, from very early on the interests and needs of the children in Norway played an important role in the process of conceptualising policies concerning children and families. The characteristic of the Norwegian welfare state as a proponent of the social democratic welfare regime, above all its universalism, makes it relatively easy to include children into the policy agenda (cf. Greve, 2000; Hemmerling, 2007; Risa, 1999; Wagner, 2006). During the period of welfare state expansion after World War II generous financial transfers for children and families as well as the expansion of the public school system took centre stage. The Norwegian welfare state has aimed at guaranteeing social security, equality and an adjustment of life chances for all members of society – including children.

When it comes to material provision for children and families, taxes and child benefits certainly have to be mentioned. Like in many other countries, the Norwegian welfare state uses the tax system to redistribute resources between families with and without children. A variety of child-related tax deductions were established. However, tax deductions tend to produce unintended effects in the sense that privileged population groups profit more from them than poorer groups. For this reason, in 1970, Norway replaced child-related tax deductions with child benefits (cf. Skevik & Hatland, 2008, p. 102).

Consequently, today child benefits are the most important financial provision for families and children. In 2005 the amount of the child benefit was 970 NOK (approx. 120€) per month and those living in the arctic regions were eligible for an additional 320 NOK (approx. 40€) for every child. The additional benefit for single parents of children aged 1–3 was 660 NOK (approx. 83€) per month (cf. Skevik & Hatland, 2008, pp. 102f). There has been effectively no increase in the child benefit since the early 1990s. At the very least, this constancy is a result of increasing the age to be included as a "child" from 16 to 18 in 2000, the financial burdens that emerged from the expansion of public childcare and the introduction of the cash-for-care benefit. In other words, a redistribution of wealth as a result of social benefits for children and families is widely accepted by the Norwegian population.

Public Daycare for Children in Norway

Given the Norwegian welfare state's longstanding stance toward the needs of children it is all the more surprising to find that the expansion of public daycare in Norway was implemented much more slowly than in many other European countries – especially compared to the other Scandinavian nations, Denmark and Sweden. Until the 1970s public daycare was mainly a phenomenon of the big cities; 80% of children in public daycare lived in cities. Reasons for this include the specific geographic and climatic conditions in Norway, the dispersed settlements in the country, the late urbanisation and industrialisation as well as the traditional dominance of industries like fishing, agriculture, forestry and shipping (cf. Korsvold, 1991, pp. 230ff). Under these conditions until the late 1960s most married women stayed at home, the farm, or went into family businesses. Furthermore, for a majority of the population the climatic living conditions outside of the cities were quite difficult. Even preschool age children contributed to the family economy by doing domestic work. There was a strong belief that parents were exclusively responsible for their children, thus the family and the home were considered to be the most appropriate place for children.

As such, the first law regarding kindergartens in 1975 viewed daycare as institutions providing an appropriate environment for children and thus must operate very closely with the parents. The task and aim of the kindergartens were oriented toward the needs of children and pedagogical concepts; other rationales like gender equality or a better reconciliation of family and work were at best seen as secondary.

Under pressure from the increased participation of females in the labour market as well as the processes of industrialisation and urbanisation, politicians negotiated the "Norwegian compromise" (cf. Korsvold, 1991) regarding the rationale of the kindergartens. Given the fact that there was a sceptical orientation towards non-familial childcare, on the one hand, and an increasing proportion of working mothers who were dependent on a sufficient supply of public childcare, on the other, kindergartens were conceived as institutions that were directly oriented toward the needs of the children. Given the specific Norwegian construction of childhood and children this means that kindergartens had to support the development of the child by enabling free play and social learning as well as by considering the individual needs of each child (cf. Strand, 2006). Everyday life in public kindergartens should approximate as closely as possible the family life and the traditional lifestyle of Norwegian children at home and should offer opportunities to spend time and play in nature.

The Ambivalence of the Norwegian Policy Concerning Children and Families

Generally speaking, all of the Scandinavian countries are considered proponents of the social democratic welfare regime type in that they combine the principle of universalism with a strong emphasis on social services. However, when it comes to social services, Norway is an exceptional case. While Norway offers a generous social services package for the elderly, those services targeting children, especially under the age of three, were at that time underdeveloped (cf. Anttonen & Sipilä, 1996). The main reason for this lies in the fact that the rationale for childcare services in Norway is – as already mentioned – not conceptualised with respect to aims like gender equality or female labour market participation, but rather with respect to pedagogical aims. Nevertheless, in the late 1980s full coverage was proclaimed as a common goal for Norwegian family policy. However, the right to childcare was not introduced for two reasons. First, the political autonomy of the local governments needed to be secured. Second, the freedom of choice between the dual-earner family model and a traditional breadwinner model had to be obtainable. This can be seen as another manifestation of the fact that the Norwegian policy does not privilege a specific model of family life, but instead pursues a "dualistic family policy" model under which both models of family life are to be encouraged (Ellingsæter, 2003; also Ellingsæter & Gulbrandsen, 2007).

The result of this was that the proportion of children in public daycare in Norway increased more slowly than in Denmark or Sweden. Whereas Denmark and Sweden managed to close the "care gap" by introducing parental leave schemes and expanding public daycare, until only recently a substantial care gap existed in Norway (Ellingsæter & Gulbrandsen, 2007, p. 654). Since the late 1980s there has been a slight expansion of public daycare. Despite this, the supply did not meet the increased demand. Ellingsæter and Gulbrandsen (cf. 2007) argue that this slow expansion cannot be explained by political strategy. Instead, they consider this the result of interactive processes between supply and demand on the childcare market. Following their line of argument, the decisive factor does not involve the policies, but rather the "mothers' agency". This means that the driving factor was not so much a political strategy but the urgent demand for public daycare especially by well-educated mothers. Adding to the considerable increase in female employment since the middle of the 1980s, there was a sharp rise in the number of full-time working mothers. In contrast to this, the provision rate increased merely from 2% in the 1960s to 20% in the 1980s. When faced with an insufficient supply of public childcare in the 1980s many parents' private initiatives were implemented to compensate for this shortage (cf. Leira, Tobio, & Trifiletti, 2005). As a consequence, the hesitant policy toward public childcare gave rise to private facilities that were supported by the state. Since the middle of the 1970s there have been approximately as many private facilities as there are public. Furthermore, only since the 1980s has the percentage of full-time slots regularly increased (78% in 2005).

In the 1990s there was a strong increase in the provision rate for public childcare. Whereas in the early 1990s merely 36% of children under 6 years of age were in public childcare, by 2000 the number had climbed to 52%. However, this impressive increase does not have as much to do with the expansion of the number of slots in public childcare, but rather can be primarily attributed to the expansion of the parental leave scheme in 1993 and the lowering of the school age from 7 to 6 in 1997.

Before 1993 the duration of parental leave was 24 weeks (30 weeks at 80% of the normal wage). The parental leave reform in 1993 extended compensation to 42 weeks at full wage or 52 weeks at 80% wage (cf. Skevik & Hatland, 2008, pp. 98f). Additionally, with the lowering of the school age to 6 years an entire age cohort was taken from the market. This meant that since 1997 the political aim has been to guarantee a slot to all children between 1 and 5 years of age if the parents request one. When it comes to trends in the childcare market the increase in the number of slots during the 1990s for children over 3 years of age was significant, whereas the number of slots for children under 3 hardly increased at all.

The Cash-for-Care Reform

The goals and the rationale of the policies concerning children and families remained contested between the left- and right-wing political parties in the years that followed. Whereas the left-wing parties preferred the dual worker family model and emphasised the goal of gender equality, the right-wing parties were oriented toward the traditional breadwinner family model and the goal of optimising choice for parents (cf. Ellingsæter, 2006). The social democratic government supported the dual breadwinner model with the parental leave reform and the expansion of early childcare and education. Afterwards the centre minority government, with the help of two other right-wing parties, attempted to support choice for parents by introducing the cash-for-care reform in order to restore balance in the dualistic family policy in Norway.

This reform pursued three goals: first, allowing parents to spend more time caring for their children, second, offering families a real choice between different care arrangements, and third, the realising of a just distribution of financial transfers between families with different care arrangements (cf. Ellingsæter, 2003; Skevik & Hatland, 2008, pp. 103f; Ellingsæter, 2006). The cash-for-care benefit was launched in August 1998 for 1-year-olds and in January 1999 for 2-year-olds. All families whose children do not have an all-day slot in public daycare are eligible. The amount of the cash-for-care benefit is 3,000 NOK (approx. 400€), which corresponds to the cost of an all-day slot at a public daycare facility. The reform which was hotly contested was preceded both by controversies in the public sphere and between the politically parties. Whereas the left-wing parties feared a roll back of the progress in gender equality, the more central- and right-wing parties criticised the lack of alternatives and the lack of choice in a policy which exclusively supports the dual-earner family model.

Interestingly enough, the effects of the reform were limited. Whereas most of the parents made use of the new cash-for-care benefit, there were only very small changes in the patterns of labour market participation by mothers. A study that was conducted shortly after the introduction of the reform showed that 1 year later just as many mothers with children between the ages of 1 and 2 were unemployed as before the reform – namely 25 or 26% – and the average weekly working hours of mothers decreased only slightly from 23.9 to 22.4 hours (cf. Ellingsæter, 2003, p. 426). Furthermore, there were no discernable effects of the reform regarding fathers. Ellingsæter found that there are no simple causal effects in the complex field of social practises within families, and that financial incentives sometimes have unintended consequences. Furthermore, family policy measures like the cash-for-care reform promote a wide variety of aims, some of which conflict to varying degrees with one another. For example, with the cash-for-care reform the choice with respect to different family models should be secured while simultaneously making it possible for parents (most often mothers) to spend more time with their children. Furthermore, a clear separation between working- and non-working mothers was assumed. On the contrary, the orientations of mothers are much more complex, and this means that many mothers combine full-time and part-time work over the course of their lives.

Since the labour market situation in Norway for mothers at the time of the reform was very good and mothers' interest in gainful employment and non-familial daycare was on the rise, mothers did not use the cash-for-care benefit to stay at home, but to pay for childcare facilities in a tight private market. Nearly one decade after the introduction of the cash-for-care benefit there is a sharp decline in the percentage of parents who make use of the benefit. The percentage went down from 74.8% of parents with children between the ages of 1 and 2 in 1999 to 47.8% by the end of 2006 – a decrease of 27% (cf. Ellingsæter & Gulbrandsen, 2007, p. 661). To a certain extent this decline was caused by the expansion of slots in public daycare for these age groups. The reform caused an opposite effect with respect to the demand for public daycare: whereas directly after the introduction of the reform the percentage of 1 and 2 year-olds in public daycare briefly declined, today the patronage of public daycare is higher than before the reform took effect and the demand is still rising. Estimates show that the percentage of children in these age groups in public daycare increased from 37% in 1999 to 62% in 2006 (cf. Ellingsæter & Gulbrandsen, 2007, p. 662).

Furthermore, the demand for public daycare increased even more as a result of the price reform in 2003. The introduction of an upper limit for public daycare costs led to a reduction in financial burdens for parents, and this, in turn, lead to even more demand for spots in public daycare.

With respect to supply and demand in the field of public daycare, it can be said that in the meantime the traditional scepticism of the Norwegian population toward public daycare has diminished. It should be noted that the high quality of the public daycare has also played a role in its increasing acceptance in Norway. Public daycare institutions are strictly controlled, there are clear norms for pedagogical quality, good staff/child ratios, and suitable surroundings. Overall, parents have a great deal of trust in the public daycare system and prefer public daycare centres to all other forms of childcare (like family centres, child minders, nannies, etc.). For this reason Ellingsæter and Gulbrandsen (cf. 2007) argue that the dynamic development in the field of public daycare in recent times is caused by the "mothers' agency" factor – this means by the extremely close interrelationship between demand and supply.

In 2003 a new political initiative changed the situation. The government and the opposition reached an agreement both on reducing the price of places in the daycare centre and at the same time offer a place to anyone who wanted to make use of daycare centres. As a consequence there was an expansion as never before in small children's enrolment at childcare centres and a subsequent reduction in use of the cash-for-care benefit. In the following years the close connection between female work participation and use of childcare centres was weakened. According to Gulbrandsen (cf. 2009), this agreement turned the relation between the supply of public subsidised daycare and mother's agency around. So far the pressures had come from well-educated mothers in the workforce. After the reform all political parties including the parties of the centre and the right wing supported the aim of guaranteeing places in public daycare for everyone who asks for it. In some sense this can be interpreted as a radical political change. However, this radical political change is not a result of a coherent political concept or strategy but is more an unintended consequence of negotiations between political parties under conditions of party competition.

However, it remains to be explained why the development in the field of child and family policies in Norway was – at least till the recent past – much more continuous than in Germany with its long period of political blockade and its recent "political revolution"? The reason as to why the development in the field of child and family policies was so steady and slow also remains unclear. The answer seems to be that the strong party cleavages in Norway prevented an overcoming of the traditional political discourses and ideas, and thus the establishment of a new cognitive and normative reference system and interpretation of external challenges and problems. Accordingly, Ellingsæter (cf. 2007) demonstrates that state interventions, as a reaction to increasing female employment and the development of new needs, are becoming increasingly complex, more diverse, and are producing new policy mixes. These complex policy packages rest on different normative rationales and ideologies. For example, measures like parental leave schemes, Daddy quota, and the expansion of public daycare are legitimised by the principle of gender equality. The intent of the Daddy quota is to help redistribute the care-giving time between mothers and fathers so that it is possible for both of them to participate in gainful employment as well as in raising children. The aim is – in the same sense as public daycare – to support the dual-earner/dual-carer family model. Contrary to this, the aim of the cash-for-care benefit is to promote the principle of choice. The goal of these measures is to give parents the opportunity to implement "good childcare", and elevate the perceived value of parental care in the society. This will be fostered by providing a choice as well as by obtaining a just distribution of financial transfers between those parents who make use of public childcare and those who do not. Although measures like this are introduced in a gender-neutral manner, the implicit rationale is to support the traditional breadwinner model. In the Norwegian party system these different policy paradigms are heavily debated and are most likely irreconcilable. Coalitions led by the social democrats tend to support the adult-worker family model, whereas the politically right-wing and centre parties adhere to measures and programs promoting choice which means that they continue to believe that the best place for children is at home.

Furthermore, in Norway there are significant obstacles impeding the introduction of a "radical social investment revolution". In this particular context there are two relevant reasons. First, the rationale of investing in the human capital – especially that of children – influenced policies both in Norway and other Scandinavian countries much earlier than in countries with a liberal or conservative welfare regime. However, these investment-oriented policies were balanced by the equally strong orientation toward the principles of security and equality. Second, the specific Norwegian interpretation of the aim of public kindergartens made sure that the principle of social investment was balanced by the strong commitment to children's needs and rights. Whereas in many countries, including Germany, efficiency-oriented learning, cognitive stimulation and school readiness are increasingly gaining support and influence in pedagogical concepts of early childcare and education, the influence of these or similar concepts in Norwegian kindergartens is thus far rather weak. As noted previously, kindergartens in Norway are designed to be safe and stimulating environments for children. Whereas free play and social learning take centre stage, education and school preparation play a relatively minor role. Nilsen (cf. 2008) and Kjorholt (cf. 2005) have extensively analysed the tight knit relationships existing between the dominating social construction of a "good childhood" as it relates to the pedagogical concepts, and the daily life in Norwegian kindergartens.

Italy: No Shift in Child and Family Policies

General Features of the Italian Welfare State

The needs and interests of children, women and families play no central role in the Italian welfare state regime; a situation attributable to its "ambivalent familism" (Saraceno, 1994). The Italian welfare state assigns the responsibilities of securing the material well-being of dependent family members to the extended family without providing much in the way of public support and care. As such, it is the family which is the de facto "key welfare provider" with an important share of both material and non-material intra-familial transfers.

Like other Mediterranean welfare states Italy represents a kind of compromise between the Bismarckian and the Beveridgian tradition (cf. Flaquer, 2000; Ferrera, 1996, 2005; Saraceno, 1997; Trifiletti, 1999). It is characterised by its high degree of fragmentation along occupational lines. As in other "Bismarckian" countries, Italy's income maintenance is based on occupational status. The degree of institutional fragmentation is easily discernable given the different schemes for private employees, civil servants and the self-employed, combined with different regulations concerning contributions and benefits. As a consequence the social security system shows a high degree of polarisation: whereas population groups working in the irregular labour market, in small firms or that are self employed are practically not covered by any social provision, population groups who work in the core sectors of the labour market or in the public sector are covered by generous social provision – especially with regard to pensions. This fragmented system of income security is flanked by a universalist health service that, since 1978, has been guarantying health care as a right of all citizens. Additionally, the Italian welfare state has no national statutory minimum income scheme. Apart from some regional programs there is no national last-resort safety net. Furthermore, there are only rudimentary indications of an explicit policy concerning children and families. To sum up, it could be stated that the Italian welfare state "is characterised not only by a preference for income transfers (particularly in the form of pensions) over transfers in kind, by a 'dualistic' protection system that makes a sharp distinction between insiders and outsiders, and by a marginal role for policies aimed directly at supporting the family (...) the family, through its gender division of labour and its intergenerational solidarity, is on the contrary expected to provide all the protection and support that is not given by a welfare state heavily biased towards pensioners and core workers" (Naldini & Saraceno, 2008, p. 734).

Family Policy Measures

As mentioned before, in Italy direct provisions for children and families – similar to other Mediterranean welfare states – are relatively underdeveloped, for example there is no universal child benefit (cf. Naldini, 2000). This does not mean, however, that policy measures aimed at children and families are non-existent. During Mussolini's rule a family allowance was introduced in 1934 in order to reach the pro-natalist objectives of the fascist regime. The family allowance went beyond the nuclear family and included dependent family members like parents, parents-in-law, and other extended relatives. After the collapse of the fascist regime and the introduction of democracy the family allowance was released from its pro-natalist aims without changing its original institutional form. The only relevant change was the extension of the provision to other social groups (e.g. the unemployed and pensioners) and to the agricultural sector. Consequently, the number of family allowance recipients continued to increase until 1974 and the associated costs also rose until 1970.

Since that time, the relevance of the family allowances in Italy has diminished drastically in terms of their real value for recipients, their share of total expenditures as a percentage of GDP, and with regard to total social expenditures (cf. Naldini, 2000, p. 73). The family allowances lost their political support because the increasingly influential unions were more interested in pension reform and in supporting the work-oriented interests of male workers than supporting families raising their children. As a result the family allowances became less important both economically and politically speaking, and that meant that the first substantial reform was implemented as late as 1988 (cf. Fargion, 2010).

The actual reform in 1988 – the initial steps for which were taken in 1983 – completely re-structured the law pertaining to the family allowance. This reform abolished family allowances and established the "household allowance" as a means-tested measure for low-income families. The new household allowance varies according to the total income of the family and the number of family members. Allowances for children are paid until 18 years of age. However, the amount of the new allowances remains fairly small. For lone-parent families and families with a disabled child or a grown-up child with a mental or physical handicap this represents a very modest increase in the household allowance. Like the original family allowance the new allowance not only covers families with children but also families with other dependent family members. Thus, it is not intended as a means of horizontal distribution between family households with and without children but as a means-tested benefit aimed at keeping low-income families from falling into poverty. The 1988 reform can be interpreted as a typical Italian-style compromise: the compromise points to a balance between the work-based social policy model of the communist party, on the one hand, and the preference of the Christian Democrats for a social assistance measure, on the other. Since the socialist party was part of the Centre Left coalitions during the 1990s the further development of child benefit was under discussion. Above all, issues like whether such a benefit should be universal or selective, means-tested or not, as well as whether it should be provided in the form of tax deductions or as a direct financial provision were discussed. However, until this day, the coalitions have not been successful in implementing a profound improvement of the system of direct financial provision for children and families.

Despite the difficulties surrounding the improvement of families and children policies, with the help of the Catholic Party in 1971 a relatively generous maternity leave program was implemented (cf. Saraceno, 1994; Menniti, Palomba, & Sabbadini, 1997). Under this program mothers receive a paid leave 2 months before the expected delivery date, for the period between the expected and actual delivery dates, and 3 months after delivery of the child (80% of their normal earnings). Maternity benefits depend on the salary of the working woman; self-employed working mothers are not eligible. Following the maternity leave, either parent (fathers since 2000) are eligible for a 1-year paid parental leave calculated as 30% of their normal income (cf. Naldini & Saraceno, 2008, pp. 740f). Working fathers of new born children are individually – and no longer only in substitution of the mother – entitled to parental leave (10 months in total until the child reaches the age of eight, of which neither parent may take more than 6 months). If the father takes at least 3 months of leave, then he is entitled to an additional month. This law has strengthened gender equality by making men's responsibilities and rights with respect to childcare more closely approximate those of women. At the same time, the flexibility with which the leave may be used has been extended; i.e. by introducing the right to take the leave for single days or only a few days a week. Yet, the effects of this law remain limited. For instance, according to recent surveys the behaviour of fathers did not change very much (cf. Naldini & Saraceno, 2008, p. 740). Furthermore, due to changes in the labour market and the increase in non-standard employment contracts, the number of workers not covered by the new provision has increased.

Public Childcare Centres and Preschools in Italy

As in other Mediterranean welfare states in Italy childcare is a family matter – or to put it more precisely: a matter for adult married women (cf. Conti & Sgritta, 2004). The issue of the division of the responsibility of caring for children between state and families is highly controversial. This situation has primarily resulted from the diametrical opposition of the ideas of the Catholic Church on the nature of the family, on the one hand, and the ideas of the political Left, on the other. As a consequence a public system of childcare – especially for children under the age of three – is extremely underdeveloped. No more than circa. 11% of children in this age group are enrolled in non-familial childcare centres. Paradoxically, in the late 1960s Italy was successful in developing a comprehensive system of preschool institutions as part of the public educational system that are now used by nearly 100% of all children between the ages of three and six. This is the reason why the dynamic expansion of Italian preschools has been called a "success story" (Della Sala, 2002, p. 182).

Public Preschools

In Italy during the early 1960s the debate over state-run preschools was quite controversial (see Della Sala, 2002; Hohnerlein, 2009). Prior to the introduction of
state preschools in 1968, the existing non-state childcare institutions were run by
Catholic orders, whose staff consisted exclusively of female teachers and assistants.
Catholic groups considered any political initiatives to increase the number of state-
run institutions, to permit male teachers and to professionalise the staff in childcare
institutions as a threat to their traditional domain. Consequently, despite the support
of the then in power Aldo Moro government, a bill introduced in 1964 proposing
state preschools failed in parliament. This was the first time in Italian history that a
government resigned due to a conflict in educational policies. This incident, however, only meant the postponement of the fundamental shift in childcare policies.
The political constellation changed with the rise of the Socialist Party as a new political actor. Later when the third Centre Left Coalition again under Aldo Moro came
into power in 1968 the new bill on state preschools[3] successfully passed the Italian
parliament. Moreover, just 1 year later the curriculum for preschools was revised
and the non-binding curriculum highlighted the pedagogical aim of focussing on
the real needs of children. At first glance the new law represents no sharp break
with the past because existing structures were not eliminated but rather flanked by
new ones. Although a political compromise, the new law nevertheless marked the
start of a far-reaching process of modernising the existing system of early childcare
and education.

The main purpose of the new preschools was the education and preparation of
children for the compulsory elementary school. Here, the role of the family was
not to be replaced but merely complemented. Enrolment in the schools was voluntary, free and offered childcare for at least 7 hours/day. The only exception to
the latter was in the South and on the Isles, where shorter opening hours were permitted. Furthermore, transportation to and from the schools as well as medical and
social care were guaranteed. A new system of financing was introduced, costs for
buildings, equipment and play material were covered by the state, and finally local
governments were responsible for costs associated with the staff, maintenance of
the buildings, heating and other running costs. Public financing is not restricted to
state-run preschools but includes private schools including schools run by religious
orders.

As mentioned before, the introduction of preschools caused a general shift in the
field of early childcare and education. This is at least due to the fact that preschools
were not defined as social services for parents (which usually meant mothers) but
as educational institutions. As such, the highly controversial issue of family responsibilities was left untouched. Furthermore, the introduction of preschools was not
legitimised by common rationales like reconciliation of family and work or pro-
natalist aims (cf. Della Sala, 2002, p. 176). Instead, the introduction of preschools
was part of the Centre Left coalition's broader aim to modernise the Italian welfare

---

[3] The Italian term for preschools in this law is "scuola maternal" (maternal schools).

state (cf. Hohnerlein, 2009, p. 98; Della Sala, 2002, p. 176). Although the central focus of the preschools was on education, political actors clearly realised the potential of the schools in achieving other social political aims. For instance, the program meant that children from poor families were provided with daily meals and health care.

In the decades that followed qualitative improvements were implemented by further legislation. Working conditions for teachers, for example, were improved by reducing the number of working hours and work load (1973), replacing the assistants with a second teacher in each class (1978), allowing male teachers to work at preschools (1983) and finally the professionalisation of the staff developed (1991/1992).

In the period from 1968 to the early 1980s there was a substantial increase in the number of children attending preschools. Whereas in the school year prior to the reform (1968/1969) 50.8% of children of the relevant age group were enrolled in non-familiar childcare institutions (95.2% of the slots were provided by non-state preschools), in 1979/1980 already 76% of the children between the ages of three to six were enrolled (60% of slots were provided by non-state preschools). At present, nearly all children – irrespective of social background and familial situation – are voluntarily enrolled in preschools, of which more than 80% are state-run (cf. Hohnerlein, 2009, p. 100 see also Naldini & Saraceno, 2008, p. 741). Starting with the 1986/1987 school year, more than 50% of preschools were state-run because many municipal and some private preschools were transformed into state-run schools for financial reasons. Whereas state-run preschools are free and only charge fees for meals and school transport, municipal fees vary according to local political decisions. In the remaining institutions the amount of the fees is directly related to the income of the parents, except the poorest parents who are not required to pay. The same also holds true for private religious preschools.

While in the field of social services – and this includes childcare centres for children under 3 years of age – the availability, number of institutions as well as the quality varies greatly from region to region, the quantitative expansion of the preschools and their spread over Italy has led to a significant reduction in the existing regional disparities compared to childcare centres and other social care services.

Childcare Centres

In stark contrast to the success of the preschools, the provision of childcare centres for children under three is still rather meagre. In Italy childcare centres belong to the system of social services. The central government's influence on the spread, quality and provision standards is quite limited. This situation is at least in part the result of the complex funding arrangement for daycare centres for which the central government is only responsible for a small part of the financial budget. The lions share comes from the block grants which the central government pays out to the regions. The regional governments pass the cost along to the municipalities either as funds specifically allocated for nurseries or through general grants to local authorities. As such, decisions concerning the financing of daycare centres are spread over different levels of government and in a near absence of binding national standards. Consequently, the provision of daycare centres varies significantly between regions – which also means a corresponding fluctuation in fees for the centres. Thus, no profound national strategy to develop a system of childcare services for children under the age of three currently exists. Adding to the difficulties is the fact that regional and local preferences regarding the quality and opening hours of local daycare facilities are often overshadowed by economic developments, financial funds and certain political constellations of actors.

Although the central government has made several attempts to develop a national childcare strategy, the fragmented structure of the political system up till now impeded any attempt to reduce persisting regional disparities. For instance, in 1971 a 5-year-plan was announced to increase the number of childcare facilities from less than 1,000 to over 3,800 as well as to enhance public administration and funding. The central government was commissioned to provide the equivalent of 0.1% of employer contributions to the Institute for Social Securities' fund to the regional governments to finance daycare centres (cf. Della Sala, 2002, pp. 177f; see also Bimbi & Della Sala, 2001). Against the backdrop of this admittedly complex financing structure it should come as no surprise that in 1976 a mere 1,080 and 10 years later no more than 1,964 daycare centres were up and running; a far cry from the originally projected 3,800 facilities by 1976. In the 1990s the number of daycare facilities stabilised to approx. 2,100 (cf. Della Sala, 2002, p. 178). As we can discern from these figures the number of children in daycare centres remained relatively low. In 1963, 2.2% of children under the age of three were enrolled in childcare centres; the percentage decreased slightly to 2.1% in 1976 and increased to 5.2% in 1986. Currently, the figure is around 11%. However, it should be noted that the regional variation is quite significant (cf. Della Sala, 2002; see also Fargion, 2010).

In Italy during the 1970s and 1980s the participation rate of woman in the labour market increased. One consequence of this development was that the preschools, which were originally intended as educational institutions, were increasingly seen as childcare institutions enabling mothers to work; a trend also acknowledged by the government. This change at the political level is reflected in the fact that within the context of the evaluation process things like the opening hours of preschools (including Saturdays) were introduced as one indicator of quality. However, a financial improvement in the support of nurseries for children under three did not follow. On the contrary, against the backdrop of the public budget crisis in the mid-1980s, the government defined childcare centres as demand-driven services which meant that daycare was transformed into a market good. This, in turn, legitimated the shifting of the burden of the higher costs to local governments and parents. While this was partly compensated for by providing greater tax deductions, the selective nature of services to be paid for by local governments and parents was nevertheless underlined. This tendency was further strengthened by the fact that in 1988 the central government transformed conditional grants into block grants. Under these conditions regional governments had to make difficult decisions regarding the programs they intended to support given their smaller budgets. Thus, day nurseries had to compete for financing with a wide variety of other social services. This meant that regions such as Calabria and Sicily, which traditionally placed childcare centres low on their list of priorities, now allocated even fewer resources to this service. The integration of different sorts of social services into one institution (i.e. combining childcare centres with preschools) or transferring certain tasks to non-governmental organisations were the outcome of new forms of rationalisation at the local level. The number of institutions of this kind, were increased. The percentage of the budget allocated to daycare centres for which the parents are responsible was increased from 11.8 to 15%.

To quickly summarise, as a consequence of the decentralisation of decision-making power both a further fragmentation of the social right to services and a further lag of coordination and coherence took place. The main result was that families – especially working mothers – were left to deal with the difficulties of balancing work and family. Empirical studies in different Italian regions demonstrate that families have been looking at private solutions to this problem. Grandmothers – resp. grandparents – were cited as the most important supporting institution in the field of childcare (cf. Naldini & Saraceno, 2008, pp. 745f). A recent empirical study confirms that only in Italy the availability of grandmothers has a slight statistical influence on the participation of women in the labour market (cf. Blome, Keck, & Alber, 2008). However, as Naldini and Saraceno (2008, pp. 745f) have pointed out this informal solution does not represent a promising future prospect. Since the next generation of women will be engaged in the labour market to a greater degree than the previous generations and as the retirement age rises, the potential reserve of care givers will shrink or will only be available at a later point, i.e. once they do actually retire. Under such conditions the conflict between the demands of the elderly in need of care and those of the younger generation will become more and more urgent.

Recent Trends in Policies Concerning Children and Families

Looking back it is clear that the Centre-Left coalitions from 1992 to 1995 as well as the Prodi government from 1996 to 2001, for the first time, tried to implement new priorities by focusing on the interests and needs of children and women as well as the previously marginal field of social services. However, these initiatives were not able to bring about a real political shift. With his return to political power in 2007 – after the Berlusconi government (2001–2006) – Prodi had a second chance to promote this ambitious endeavour. In fact, it was during this administration that for the first time a Minister of Family Affairs was established. The new Minister, Rosy Bindi, was even able to introduce several political initiatives moving in this direction, for example a 3-year plan to expand childcare services. A total of 770 million Euro was provided to create 40,000 new slots for children aged 0–2 as well as a further 24,000 slots for children aged 2–3 in the period from 2007 to 2009. With this target the Prodi government was far below the Centre-Left electoral commitment to guarantee 100,000 new slots as well as the Barcelona target of 33%

coverage (cf. Fargion, 2010). Additionally, an annual tax deduction of up to 632€ was launched to help cover the cost of public and private childcare institutions. However, when compared to the average monthly cost of 400€ for childcare, it is obvious that this measure was completely inadequate. Furthermore, some smaller improvements to family benefits, which, in accordance with the fragmented and category-based pattern of the Italian policy-making process, only addresses specific forms of families (i.e. families with disabled dependents), are not able to change the fact that the second Prodi government was also not able to reach a profound breakthrough in the field of policies concerning children and families. This also holds true for the Berlusconi government which came into power in May 2008. However, under the current coalition personnel cuts in primary, secondary, and higher education as well as financial cutbacks involving the National Long-term Care Fund established by the previous Centre-Left coalition have rather contributed to the increased burden of women and families as well as worsen the conditions of combining work and family (cf. Fargion, 2010).

Conclusion

This chapter argues that children and families play an increasingly important role in welfare politics. In many countries, expenditures for benefits and services aimed at children and families increased or could at least be sustained despite the declining share of children in the overall population. We have witnessed over the last 10–15 years the development of new priorities in the policies concerning children and families. Nevertheless, there are considerable differences between countries. Despite the fact that all countries are more or less confronted with the same challenges, for example, an aging population, low birth rates, and structural change in the families, some countries have developed new political priorities while others have not. Obviously the development of a new political direction is not simply a reaction to a different set of external challenges. Taking Norway, Germany, and Italy as case studies, this essay has examined the relevance of political discourses and ideas in policies concerning children and families.

As the Norwegian case demonstrates policies concerning children and families in Norway have developed along a more continuous path. This is primarily attributable to the traditionally important role the interests and needs of children play in Norwegian politics. Hence, in Norway changes in political priorities and instruments can be understood as reactions to changed economic and social conditions. On the other hand, the central role of children and childhood in the Norwegian public discourse made it, in the wake of the UN-Convention, relatively easy to adapt policies to new ideas like the children's right discourse. Accordingly, the children's rights approach exerted great influence in child-oriented politics not only regarding the development of new institutions concerning the participation of children at the local level like ombudspersons, Children and Youth Parliaments, etc., but also in implementation of children's social rights in the social policy field.

Moreover, in Norway – as a proponent of the Scandinavian welfare regime – a strong expansion of the public childcare system took place without any radical changes in the ideas and discourses concerning children and family policies. Several reasons can be given for this: First, although Norway was a relative latecomer compared to countries like Sweden and Denmark in the field of expanding public childcare facilities, it was nevertheless much further along than Germany. Norway, in contrast to Germany, has already reached the Barcelona benchmark (provision rate for children under the age of three: 33%). Since the middle of the 1980s, there has been a steady increase in the number of public childcare places in Norway. This trend was driven by a high demand for female employment and a strong preference for public daycare among Norwegian mothers. Second, there was no need for a radical change in the ideas and values concerning children and families because of the strong traditional commitment of the Norwegian society to children's needs and rights. Given the relevance of children in Norwegian society as well as for the further development of Norwegian identity the investment in children has always been a traditional aim of Norwegian child policies. Consequently, and in contrast to Germany, it was not necessary to "discover" children as important citizens. Furthermore, the social construction of childhood in Norway works as an effective barrier against the influence of the new social investment ideology and the exclusive definition of children as "citizen-workers of the future".

However, policies concerning children and families underwent a profound change over the last few decades. Instead of a radical change there was, as mentioned above, a very gradual modernisation that began at the end of the 1970s. As this chapter shows, this change cannot be explained by the introduction of a new political paradigm and a new social construction of children and childhood, but by the reaction of the Norwegian state to the preferences of mothers and the increasing demand for non-familial childcare – even for very young children (mothers' agency). It was not until 2003 that a broad political agreement concerning the expansion of the public childcare system was negotiated. Since then, not only well-educated mothers but also low income families make use of public childcare. Instead of introducing a new political model of a "good childhood" and a "good family life" – like in many other countries – the normative foundation of the Norwegian policy concerning children and families remains the same. The political package for children and families in Norway is characterised by a combination of public childcare and a cash-for-care benefit combined with a relatively generous child benefit. This is both the result of a political compromise between the parties of the left, on the one hand, and the parties of the centre and the right wing, on the other (cf. Gulbrandsen, 2009). And this is the reason why the birth rate in Norway compared to other European countries is relatively high, whereas child poverty is relatively low.

In contrast to this, in Germany ideas, values and discourses played an important role in policy change. In Germany it was possible to establish a new political discourse concerning the status and role of children and families in society as well as change the interpretations of needs and preferences of influential political actors. Until recently, family policy in Germany was oriented toward the traditional male-breadwinner family model and a social construction of childhood, which interprets children as dependent parts of the private family sphere. Under these conditions family policy in Germany adhered to a policy package characterised both by a dominance of financial transfers and a deficit of social services. Consequently, Germany was, at the beginning of the twenty-first century, confronted with a backlogged demand regarding the reconciliation of family and work for working mothers and public childcare (especially for children under 3 years of age). It was under these conditions that the political actors in the Ministry of Family Affairs identified the need for a radical change. They established the new concept of a "sustainable family policy". However, in the multiple-actor system of the Federal Republic of Germany – with its distribution of power between the federal state, "Bundesländern", and local governments, not to mention the relevance of non-profit organisations – in order to achieve actual political change it is decisive to find political partners and built advocacy coalitions. This is the reason why the Ministry of Family Affairs attached such great importance to attracting influential scientific experts as supporters for both formulating and implementing the new concept of sustainable family policy as well as for building alliances with different actors from all sectors of society. The rationale underlying this concept of family policy is that investing in children is advantageous not only for children, but for society as a whole. The new policy model was presented as a comprehensive strategy of economic modernisation in order to convince both other political actors and the public, and was totally in line with the social investment approach. However, although political actors managed to implement a paradigm shift, so far the new political concept has not made a great impact. As demonstrated, no increase in the birth rate has taken place. Although the Minister of Family Affairs, Ursula von der Leyen, expected to see an increase in the fertility rate just 1 year after the reform of the parental leave program, no significant increase in the number of births was detected. The fertility rate in Germany is still one of the lowest in Europe. Furthermore, Germany was not able to reduce the child poverty rate. According to recent studies, however, the risk of poverty for children under 15 years of age (measured against the 60% threshold) increased from 15.7% in 2000 to 26.3% in 2006 (cf. Olk & Hübenthal, 2009). Additionally, the expansion of publicly financed daycare did not proceed as rapidly as the Ministry expected. An analysis shows that in order to reach the political goal of implementing a provision rate of 35% for those under 3 years of age in Western Germany by 2013 the current expansion rate needs to be doubled (cf. Bock-Famulla, 2008).

As such, Germany represents an interesting case in the field of policies concerning children and families. On the one hand, Germany is a good example for demonstrating that a profound shift in the political priorities can be implemented under the conditions of a conservative welfare regime, thus we have an alternative to the theory of path dependency. On the other hand, implementing a new paradigm in the field of child and family policies was not able to produce long-term results. This is partly due to the fact that the paradigm shift has been restricted to the Ministry of Family Affairs; other Ministries simply follow their own rationales. As a consequence, political contradictions and tensions between different political departments persist within the German government, thus hindering the establishment of a new coherent political strategy concerning children and families.

Italy, a Mediterranean welfare state, is the counterpart to Norway. In both countries (in contrast to Germany) policies concerning children and families are characterised by a strong commitment to continuity. However, whereas in Norway the orientation toward the interests and needs of children has always been strong, in Italy children and families have never been a high priority on the political agenda. The strong tradition of an "ambivalent familism" combined with the fragmented and category-based character of the political processes in Italy impeded any break-through in the policies concerning children and families. Neither the children's rights approach, nor the social investment approach has been able to gain influence in Italy's political debates and discourses. Given the Catholic Churches' conception of the nature of the family, the division of the responsibility for children between family and the state is highly controversial. Thus, in order to appease the Catholic Church the success of establishing new political priorities concerning child and family policies is dependent on not directly thematising the issue. One such prominent example is the development of a comprehensive system of preschools. The success of this project rested upon defining preschools as educational institutions rather than social services aimed at easing the burden of balancing work and family responsibilities for working mothers. Despite all efforts, it was not possible to develop an explicit family policy aimed at improving the living conditions of families with children, i.e. by means of a horizontal redistribution between family households with and without children. Instead, political measures and instruments continue to focus on preventing low income families from falling into poverty. Furthermore, a national childcare strategy capable of improving the conditions for reconciling family and work as well as improving the living conditions of children has yet to be realised. This is a somewhat paradoxical fact because the challenges facing Italy in this policy field are significant. Italy suffers from an extremely low fertility rate, a relatively high child poverty rate, and relatively poor conditions for reconciling family and work for a growing number of working mothers. The discrepancy between external challenges and the lack of political response demonstrates, however, that Italy still can not afford to release itself from the previous "old" policy oriented toward the industrial society. In other words, Italy has failed to establish a new political strategy that pushes the interests and needs of children and families higher up on the political agenda.

References

Amann, S. (2006). Wie das Elterngeld wirklich wirkt. *Spiegel Online 2009, Spiegelnet GmbH*. Retrieved from http://www.spiegel.de/wirtschaft/0,1518,623066,00.html

Anttonen, A., & Sipilä, J. (1996). European social care services: Is it possible to identity models? *Journal of European Social Policy, 6*(1), 87–100.

Bertram, H., Rösler, W., & Ehlert, N. (2005). *Nachhaltige Familienpolitik. Zukunftssicherung durch einen Dreiklang von Zeitpolitik, finanzieller Transferpolitik und Infrastrukturpolitik*. Berlin: Bundesministeriums für Familie, Senioren, Frauen und Jugend.

Bimbi, F., & Della Sala, V. (2001). Italy: Policy without participation. In J. Jenson & M. Sineau (Eds.), *Who cares? Women's work, childcare, and welfare state redesign* (pp. 118–145). Toronto: University of Toronto Press.

Blome, A., Keck, W., & Alber, J. (2008). *Generationenbeziehungen im Wohlfahrtsstaat: Lebensbedingungen und Einstellungen von Altersgruppen im internationalen Vergleich.* Wiesbaden, VS: Verlag für Sozialwissenschaften.

BMFSFJ. (2006). *Familie zwischen Flexibilität und Verlässlichkeit. Perspektiven für eine lebenslaufbezogene Familienpolitik.* Berlin: Siebter Familienbericht.

BMFSFJ. (2008, September 28). *Pressemitteilung des Bundesministeriums für Familie, Senioren, Frauen und Jugend zum Kinderförderungsgesetz* (KiföG), Berlin.

Bock-Famulla, K. (2008). *Länderreport Frühkindliche Bildungssysteme.* Gütersloh: Bertelsmann Stiftung.

Conti, C., & Sgritta, G. B. (2004). Childhood in Italy: A family affair. In A. M. Jensen, A. Ben-Arieh, C. Conti, D. Kutsar, M. N. Ghiolla Phádraig, & H. Warming Nilsen (Eds.), *Children's welfare in ageing Europe* (Vol. 1, pp. 81–142). Trondheim: Norwegian Centre for Child Research.

Della Sala, V. (2002). Modernization and welfare-state restructuring in Italy: The impact on child care. In S. Michel & R. Mahon (Eds.), *Child care policy at the crossroads: Gender and welfare state restructuring* (pp. 171–190). London: Routledge.

Dobrowolsky, A., & Jenson, J. (2005). Social investment perspectives and practices: A decade in British politics. *Social Policy Review, 17,* 203–230.

Ellingsæter, A. L. (2003). The complexity of family policy reform. The case of Norway. *European Societies, 5*(4), 419–443.

Ellingsæter, A. L. (2006). The Norwegian childcare regime and its paradoxes. In A. L. Ellingsæter (Ed.), *Politicising parenthood in Scandinavia. Gender relations in welfare states* (pp. 121–144). Cambridge: The Policy Press.

Ellingsæter, A. L. (2007). 'Old' and 'new' politics of time to care: Three Norwegian reforms. *Journal of European Social Policy, 17*(49), 49–60.

Ellingsæter, A. L., & Gulbrandsen, L. (2007). Closing the childcare gap: The interaction of childcare provision and mothers' agency in Norway. *Journal of Social Policy, 36*(4), 649–669.

Esping-Andersen, G. (1990). *The three worlds of welfare capitalism.* Cambridge: The Policy Press.

Esping-Andersen, G. (2002). A child-centred social investment strategy. In G. Esping-Andersen, D. Gallie, A. Hemerijck, & J. Myles (Eds.), *Why we need a new welfare state* (pp. 26–67). Oxford: University Press.

Esping-Anderson, G. (2005). *Children in the welfare state. A social investment approach.* DemoSoc Working Paper No. 2005–10.

Esping-Andersen, G. (2008). Childhood investments and skill formation. *International Tax and Public Finance, 15*(1), 19–44.

Fargion, V. (2010). Children, gender and families in the Italian welfare state. In J. Gal & M. Ajzenstadt (Eds.), *Gender families and children in Mediterranean welfare states.* New York: Springer:105–128.

Ferrera, M. (1996). The 'Southern Model' of welfare in social Europe. *Journal of European Social Policy, 6*(17), 17–37.

Ferrera, M. (2005). Welfare states and social safety nets in Southern Europe: An introduction. In M. Ferrera (Ed.), *Welfare state reform in Southern Europe, fighting poverty and social exclusion in Italy, Spain, Portugal and Greece* (pp. 1–32). London: Routledge.

Flaquer, L. (2000). Is there a Southern European model of family policy? In A. Pfenning & T. Bahle (Eds.), *Family and family policy in Europe: Comparative perspectives* (pp. 15–33). Frankfurt am Main: Peter Lang.

Gabel, S. G., & Kamerman, S. B. (2006). *Investing in children: Public commitment in twenty-one industrialized countries in social review.* Chicago: The University of Chicago.

Greve, B. (2000). Family policy in the Nordic countries. In A. Pfenning & T. Bahle (Eds.), *Families and family policy in Europe: Comparative perspectives* (pp. 90–103). Frankfurt am Main: Peter Lang.

Gulbrandsen, L. (2009). The Norwegian cash-for-care reform: Changing behaviour and stable attitudes. *Nordisk Barnehageforskning, 2*(1), 17–25.

Hall, P. A. (1993). Policy paradigms, social learning, and the state: The case of economic policymaking in Britain. *Comparative Politics, 25*(3), 275–296.

Hemmerling, A. (2007). *Der Kindergarten als Bildungsinstitution. Hintergründe und Perspektiven.* Wiesbaden, VS: Verlag für Sozialwissenschaften.

Hohnerlein, E. M. (2009). The paradox of public preschools in a familist welfare regime: The Italian case. In K. Scheiwe & H. Willekens (Eds.), *Child care and preschool development in Europe: Institutional perspectives* (pp. 88–104). Houndmills: Palgrave Macmillan.

James, A., & James, A. L. (2004). *Constructing childhood: Theory, policy and social practice.* Houndmills: Palgrave Macmillan.

James, A., & James, A. L. (2005). Introduction: The politics of childhood – An overview. In J. Goddard, S. McNamee, A. James, & A. L. James (Eds.), *The politics of childhood. International perspectives, contemporary developments* (pp. 3–12). Houndmills: Palgrave Macmillan.

Jenson, J. (2004). Changing the paradigm: Family responsibility or investing in children. *The Canadian Journal of Sociology, 29*(2), 169–192.

Jenson, J., & Saint-Martin, D. (2003). New routes to social cohesion? Citizenship and the social investment state. *Canadian Journal of Sociology, 28*(1), 77–99.

Jurczyk, K., Olk, T., & Zeiher, H. (2004). German children's welfare between economy and ideology. In A. M. Jensen, A. Ben-Arie, C. Conti, D. Kutsar, M. Ghiolla Phádraig, & H. W. Nielsen (Eds.), *Children's welfare in ageing Europe* (Vol. 2, pp. 703–770). Trondheim: Norwegian Center for Child Research.

Kjorholt, A. T. (2005). The competent child and the 'right to be oneself': Reflections on children as fellow citizens in an early childhood centre. In A. Clark, A. Kjorholt, & P. Moss (Eds.), *Beyond listening: Children's perspectives on early children's services* (pp. 151–175). Bristol: Policy Press.

Korsvold, T. (1991). Kindergarten und Kulturvermittlung. Entwicklung und Eigenarten des norwegischen Kindergarten-Modells. *Pädagogische Rundschau, 45*(2), 227–237.

Kuebler, D. (2007). Understanding the recent expansion of Swiss family policy: An idea-centred approach. *Journal of Social Policy, 36*(2), 217–237.

Leira, A., Tobio, C., & Trifiletti, R. (2005). Kinship and informal support: Care resources for the first generation of working mothers in Norway, Italy and Spain. In U. Gerhard, T. Knijn, & A Weckwert (Eds.), *Working mothers in Europe: A comparison of policies and practices* (pp. 74–96). Cheltenham: Edward Elgar.

Leitner, S. (2008). Ökonomische Funktionalität der Familienpolitik oder familienpolitische Funktionalisierung der Ökonomie. In A. Evers & R. G. Heinze (Eds.), *Sozialpolitik. Ökonomisierung und Entgrenzung* (pp. 67–82). Wiesbaden, VS: Verlag für Sozialwissenschaften.

Lister, R. (2004). The Third way's social investment state. In H. Lewis & R. Surender (Eds.), *Welfare state change: Toward a third way?* (pp. 157–181). New York: Oxford University Press.

Lister, R. (2006). An agenda for children: Investing in the future or promoting well-being in the present? In J. Lewis (Ed.), *Children, changing families and welfare states* (pp. 51–66). Cheltenham: Edward Elgar.

Menniti, A., Palomba, R., & Sabbadini, L. L. (1997). Italy: Changing the family from within. In F. X. Kaufmann, A. Kuijsten, H. J. Schulze, & K. P. Strohmeier (Eds.), *Family life and policies in Europe: Structures and trends in the 1980s* (Vol. 1, pp. 225–252). Oxford: Clarendon Press.

Mohn, L., & von der Leyen, U. (Eds.). (2007). *Familie gewinnt: die Allianz und ihre Wirkungen für Unternehmen und Gesellschaft.* Gütersloh: Bertelsmann Stiftung.

Naldini, M. (2000). Family allowances in Italy and Spain: Long ways to reform. In A. Pfenning & T. Bahle (Eds.), *Family and family policy in Europe: Comparative perspectives* (pp. 70–89). New York: Peter Lang.

Naldini, M., & Saraceno, C. (2008). Social and family policies in Italy: Not totally frozen but far from structural reforms. *Social Policy & Administration, 42*(7), 733–748.

Nilsen, R. D. (2008). Children in nature: Cultural ideas and social practices in Norway. In A. James, A. L. James (Eds.), *European childhoods: Cultures, politics and childhoods in Europe* (pp. 38–60). New York: Palgrave Macmillian.

OECD. (2001). *Starting strong: Early childhood and care*. Paris: OECD.

OECD. (2006). *Starting strong II: Early childhood education and care*. Paris: OECD.

Olk, T., & Hübenthal, M. (2009). Child poverty in the German social investment state. *Journal of Family Research, 21*(2), 150–167.

Olk, T., & Wintersberger, H. (2007). Welfare states and generational order. In H. Wintersberger, L. Alanen, T. Olk, & J. Qvortrup (Eds.), *Childhood, generational order and the welfare state: Exploring children's social and economic welfare* (Vol. 1, pp. 59–90). Odense: University Press of Southern Denmark.

Qvortrup, J. (2008). Childhood in the welfare state. In A. James & A. L. James (Eds.), *European childhoods: Cultures, politics and childhoods in Europe* (pp. 216–233). Houndmills: Palgrave Macmillan.

Rauschenbach, T. (2006). Wer betreut Deutschlands Kinder? Eine einleitende Skizze In W. Bien, T. Rauschenbach, & B. Riedel (Eds.), *Wer betreut Deutschlands Kinder? DJI-Kinderbetreuungsstudie* (pp. 10–24). Weinheim/Basel: Beltz.

Risa, A. E. (1999). Familienpolitik in Norwegen. In C. Leipert (Ed.), *Aufwertung der Erziehungsarbeit. Europäische Perspektiven einer Strukturreform der Familien- und Gesellschaftspolitik* (pp. 245–258). Opladen: Leske und Budrich.

Ristau, M. (2005). Der ökonomische Charme der Familie. In Aus Politik und Zeitgeschichte (ApuZ). *Beilage zur Zeitschrift Das Parlament, 23–24*, 16–23.

Rürup, B., & Gruesco, S. (2003). *Nachhaltige Familienpolitik im Interesse einer aktiven Bevölkerungsentwicklung: Gutachten im Auftrag des Bundesministeriums für Familie, Senioren, Frauen und Jugend*. Berlin: Bundesministerium für Familie, Senioren, Frauen und Jugend.

Saraceno, C. (1994). The ambivalent familism of the Italian welfare state. *Social Politics, 1*(1), 60–82.

Saraceno, C. (1997). Family change, family policies and the restructuring of welfare. In OECD (Ed.), *Family, market and community: Equity and efficiency in social policy* (pp. 81–100). Paris: OECD Social Policy Studies 21.

Satka, M., & Eydal, G. B. (2004). The history of Nordic policies for children. In H. Brembeck, B. Johansson, & J. Kampmann (Eds.), *Beyond the competent child: Exploring contemporary childhood in the Nordic welfare societies* (pp. 33–61). Roskilde: Roskilde University Press.

Schmidt, V. A. (2002). Does discourse matter in the politics of welfare state adjustment? *Comparative Political Studies, 35*(2), 168–193.

Schmidt, V. A., & Radaelli, C. M. (2004). Policy change and discourse in Europe: Conceptual and methodological issues. *West European Politics, 27*(2), 183–210.

Skevik, A., & Hatland, A. (2008). Family policies in Norway. In I. Ostner & C. Schmitt (Eds.), *Family policies in the context of family change. The Nordic countries in comparative perspective* (pp. 89–107). Wiesbaden: Verlag für Sozialwissenschaften.

Sørensen, Ø., & Stråth, B. (Eds.). (1997). *The cultural construction of Norden*. Oslo, Stockholm, Copenhagen, Oxford, Boston: Scandinavian University Press.

Spieß, K. C., Berger, E. M., & Groh-Samberg, O. (2008). *Die öffentlich geförderte Bildungs- und Betreuungsinfrastruktur in Deutschland: Eine ökonomische Analyse regionaler und nutzer-gruppenspezifischer Unterschiede*. Innocenti Working Paper 2008–03. Florence: UNICEF Innocenti Research Centre.

Strand, T. (2006). The social game of early childhood education. The case of Norway. In J. Einarsdottir & J. T. Wagner (Eds.), *Nordic childhoods and early education, philosophy, research, policy, and practice in Denmark, Finland, Iceland, Norway and Sweden* (pp. 71–99). Greenwich: Information Age Publishing.

Therborn, G. (1993). The politics of childhood: The rights of children in modern times. In F. Castles (Ed.), *Families of nations: Patterns of public policy in western democracies* (pp. 241–293). Aldershot: Avebury.

Trifiletti, R. (1999). Southern European welfare regimes and the worsening position of women. *Journal of European Social Policy, 9*(1), 29–64.

Wagner, J. T. (2006). An outsider's perspectives. Childhoods and early education in the Nordic countries. In J. Einarsdottir & J. T. Wagner (Eds.), *Nordic childhoods and early education. Philosophy, research, policy, and practice in Denmark, Finland, Iceland, Norway and Sweden* (pp. 289–306). Greenwich: Information Age Publishing.

Yee, A. S. (1996). The causal effects of ideas on policies. *International Organization, 50*(1), 69–108.

Understanding Gender Economic Inequality Across Welfare Regimes

Hadas Mandel

Introduction

The process of "farewell to maternalism" (Orloff, 2006) has taken diverse forms in different societies over the last few decades. With the massive entry of women into the labor market, significant cross-country variations have emerged not only in the level of women's employment but also in their patterns of integration and in the nature of gender stratification in the labor market. To keep pace with this process, the literature on welfare states and gender stratification has branched out to cover a variety of gendered outcomes, besides women's participation rates. This variability has yielded contradictory conclusions concerning the implications of welfare states for gender stratification. While countries characterized by progressive family policies were generally found to be those with the highest women's labor market participation rates, and thus the lowest levels of women's economic dependency and poverty rates, they were also found to be those with the lowest women's occupational and earnings attainment (e.g. Daly, 2000; Esping-Andersen, 1999; Korpi, 2000; Mandel & Semyonov, 2005, 2006; Misra, Budig, & Moller, 2007; Orloff, 2006; Wright, Baxter, & Birkelund, 1995).

This chapter seeks to understand the equivocal findings of previous studies by analyzing multiple aspects of gender inequality simultaneously and mapping them into distinctive profiles. Shifting the focus from a single aspect of gender inequality to the relation between several aspects, the chapter examines the inherent tradeoffs between them, relating these tradeoffs to the institutional context in general and to welfare state strategies in particular.

The empirical evidence to illustrate the different strategies of state interventions and their relations to gender inequality are provided by four countries: Sweden, the United States, Germany, and Italy. Following Esping-Andersen's (1990) classic typology, Sweden and the USA are prime examples of the social-democratic and liberal welfare regimes, respectively, while Germany is a continental-conservative and

H. Mandel (✉)
Tel-Aviv University, Tel-Aviv, Israel
e-mail: hadasm@post.tau.ac.il

M. Ajzenstadt, J. Gal (eds.), *Children, Gender and Families in Mediterranean Welfare States*, Children's Well-Being: Indicators and Research 2, DOI 10.1007/978-90-481-8842-0_2, © Springer Science+Business Media B.V. 2010

Italy a Mediterranean-conservative country. As each of the four countries represents a different type of welfare state, I have chosen them as representative cases to establish the linkage between welfare state policy and patterns of gender inequality. Thus, after framing the institutional context in general, the distinctive pattern of gender stratification in each welfare regime will be identified, empirically illustrated, and theoretically related to the different institutional context that characterizes each regime.

The findings of this chapter reinforce the assertion that state interventions, especially the ways in which public policies encourage or repress women's entry into the labor market, have a crucial bearing on the nature of gender stratification. Moreover, the findings show that mapping multiple aspects of gender inequality and assembling them into distinctive profiles not only reveals the costs and benefits of each policy regime, but also highlights the linkage between welfare state strategies and their presumed outcomes.

Framing the Institutional Context

The most well-known contribution to the distinction between different profiles of state intervention is that of Gosta Esping-Andersen (1990). Despite, or maybe because of, the vast feminist criticism of Esping-Andersen's welfare regimes, (e.g. Gornick, Meyers, & Ross, 1997; Langan & Ostner, 1991; Lewis, 1992; O'Connor, 1993; Orloff, 1993) his threefold terminology has deeply permeated feminist research and taken up permanent residence in studies of the welfare state and gender inequality. To rebut feminist accusations of neglect of gender-related criteria and the effect of welfare state institutions on gender relations, in his 1999 book Esping-Andersen relates different modes of care provision to different welfare regimes and stresses their importance for understanding a variety of gendered outcomes, such as women's labor force participation and fertility rates. He also coined the term "defamilialism" – which describes the extent to which the state (or the market) reduces the centrality of the family as a welfare provider. As an analytical tool for analyzing the relationship between the state, the market, and the family, this term has become fundamental to any discussion of welfare regimes and gender inequality.

Subsequently, a considerable body of comparative research has largely recognized the explanatory power of Esping-Andersen's triple typology as a basis for distinguishing between institutional contexts, and its importance to gender. These studies confirm that forms of state intervention, as reflected by the provision of welfare and care services, vary significantly across welfare regimes, and therefore across the four countries that represent them in this study (e.g. Esping-Andersen, 1990, 1999; Gornick & Meyers, 2003; Korpi, 2000; Misra et al., 2007). Sweden typifies the dual-earner model, where the state takes an active role in providing social and family services; in the USA, markets are the dominant mechanism for service provision; while Germany and Italy follow what Lewis (1992) described as the "male breadwinner" model, in which the state attempts to preserve the traditional division of labor in the home and foster reliance on the family for providing both welfare and care services.

The different modes of state interventions constitute the interpretive framework of this chapter. This interpretive framework is illustrated by ideal types of welfare regimes, which explain the different patterns of gender stratification. Patterns of gender stratification are identified by multiple indicators of gender economic inequality. In order to encompass the major expressions of gender inequality, different indicators of women's economic position are utilized, from rates of labor force participation, through occupational attainments and economic rewards, to outcomes such as poverty rates and economic autonomy. This collection of indicators not only covers a wide range of women's economic positions, but also comprises measures that capture the economic position of women in different class situations (such as access to managerial positions at the top and poverty rates at the bottom). Detailed definitions of the variables and measures are found in Appendix 1.

In the following three sections I will show that the diversified indicators constitute a unique configuration of gender stratification in the four countries studied, which can be best understood by the dominant modes of state intervention in each context. Because the importance of my analysis lies in its potential for highlighting configurations rather than distinctive dimensions, cross-country comparisons will encompass several indicators presented in the different figures, and will refer to each figure several times. All figures and Table 1 are therefore located at the end of the chapter.

The Social-Democratic Context – Equal Employment, Unequal Achievements

The social-democratic welfare state advances a "dual-earner model" which, unlike the other regimes, is explicitly targeted at encouraging the employment of women. Although not its sole purpose, one of the goals of this policy is to advance gender equality by reducing women's economic dependence. The active role that the state takes in encouraging women's paid work is based on the social-democratic tradition, which sees the provision of social services on a universal basis as a primary means of promoting equality. Historically, this model can be found as early as the 1940s and 1950s, when a career woman was still an unusual phenomenon, but the idea of "women's two roles" had begun to gain momentum (Lewis, 1990). During the 1960s, with the establishment of the welfare state and the massive growth of the public services sector, the ideology of "women's two roles" was replaced with the ideology of the dual-earner family. In contrast to the former, which encouraged the incorporation of women into paid work before and after raising their small children, the dual-earner ideology supported women's entry into the labor market even when they were mothers to young children, aimed at integrating work and family throughout the life cycle. Within this ideological framework, legislation protecting social rights in general, and working mothers in particular, was formulated and institutionalized, in addition to the extension of childcare services provided by the public sector (e.g. Lewis and Astrom, 1992; Korpi, 2000; Ellingsater, 2009).

The exclusive feature of this welfare regime is not its emphasis on the importance of employment as a means of attaining gender equality, but rather its translation into practical terms. This is demonstrated by the large supply of public daycares subsidized by the state, in addition to the use of the public sector as a mechanism for creating jobs for women (Esping-Andersen, 1990). Because of the active role of the state as an employer, most working women in social-democratic countries operate within a protected labor market, which provides them with flexible terms of employment while protecting their rights as mothers. Other universal benefits and entitlements that protect mothers come in the form of lengthy maternity leave and job security.

Figure 1 provides data on female labor force participation that affirm the efficiency of the Swedish dual-earner model in raising women's participation rates, most notably among mothers of young children (see also Daly, 2000; Gornick et al., 1997; Korpi, 2000; Mandel & Semyonov, 2006). The success of the Swedish model in raising women's participation rates is also revealed by the prevalence of dual-earner households, and the tiny proportion of couple-headed households in which the male is the sole earner, as shown in Fig. 2.

The fact that the Swedish state allows women easy access to an independent income increases their economic contribution to the household at a significantly higher rate than in the other countries, and thus reduces their economic dependency on their partners, as seen in Fig. 3. Earnings dependency is measured by the gap (in favor of the husband/partner) between the relative contributions of the two spouses to the household income (see also Bianchi, Casper, & Peltola, 1999). In the gray bar – which displays dependency level by earnings alone – dependency levels are primarily influenced by access to a paycheck, although they also reflect differences between the spouses' incomes. The black bar – which displays dependency level after adding childcare and maternity allowances to women's contribution – indicates that state generosity towards mothers in Sweden further reduces women's dependency levels. This, however, does not inhibit their high rates of paid employment.

The high proportion of working mothers not only reduces women's economic dependence on their spouses' income, but also enables women to make a living without relying on a spouse's salary at all. The empirical evidence for this is provided by the relatively low poverty rates among single mothers in Sweden, as shown in Table 1 (see also, Christopher, 2002; Kilkey & Bradshaw, 1999; Casper, McLanahan, & Garfinkel, 1994). Poverty rates among both working and nonworking single mothers are relatively low, and almost half of the single mothers in Sweden are single, compared to only 4% who are widows. This implies that single motherhood in Sweden is often a matter of choice, one that is made possible by the state's support for single mothers.

The impressive entry of Swedish women into the labor market and the relative economic autonomy they enjoy from their partners have not, however, been accompanied by equality of labor market attainments. On the contrary, in the protected Swedish labor market women are more concentrated in female-type jobs within the public sector, and, compared to other countries, have less access to positions of power and prestige and enjoy lower economic rewards (e.g. Mandel & Semyonov, 2006; Wright et al., 1995). Figures 4 and 5 illustrate this through two of the most notable parameters of gender inequality in Scandinavian countries – horizontal and vertical gender segregation. Compared to the other three countries, Sweden has the highest rate of occupational sex segregation and the lowest proportion of women in managerial positions. Given the high rewards that usually accompany these positions and the comparatively low pay typical of female-type occupations, women's position in the occupational structure has tangible consequences for their economic achievements (Petersen & Morgan, 1995). Figure 6 shows the proportion of women in each country's top and bottom wage quintiles. Sweden is the country farthest removed from egalitarian representation – 20% – at both poles of the wage structure. Women are overrepresented in the bottom quintile and underrepresented at the top.

It would appear, then, that equality in Sweden, as represented by employment yardsticks, reverts to inequality when measured by labor market achievements. While the social-democratic state does succeed in bringing more women into the work cycle, it places them in a "feminine niche" that provides them with comfortable working conditions, but at an economic and social price. The comfortable terms of employment enable women to be both workers and caregivers, but make it more difficult for them to compete with men for high positions and economic rewards within the labor market. As many feminists claim, the massive entry of women into the labor market in social-democratic countries has not altered the traditional division of labor between men and women, but rather transferred it from the household to the labor market (e.g. Hernes, 1987; Langan & Oster, 1991; O'Connor, 1993; Orloff, 1996). My claim is that this specific pattern of gender stratification is a direct product of the dual-earner model. In other words, the very attempt to fit the labor market to women in the social-democratic regime perpetuates women's economic inferiority, because it sustains the model of "women's two roles" (worker and caregiver) as opposed to "men's one role," by sapping women's motivation to compete with men over market rewards and making female workers less attractive to employers.

The stratified configuration of the social-democratic welfare state, however, should be judged and understood within its ideological context. Although the benefits accruing to working mothers make female workers less attractive to private employers, this is a byproduct of a broader aim. Through social-democratic lenses, full employment for women – even at the price of their concentration in the public sector and exclusion from positions of power – is an important step towards equality, as it protects most women from poverty, and fulfills their right to independence: liberation from long-term dependency on their spouses and families or the state's welfare institutions. This byproduct is a reasonable price to pay in a social-democratic ideological context, which aspires to advance equality on a universal basis, even at the expense of maximizing profits for strong groups.

The Conservative Context – Unequal Employment, Equal Achievements

The social-democratic regime finds its mirror image in western and southern European states – the conservative welfare regime, according to Esping-Andersen's typology. In contrast to employment-supportive policies in social-democratic states, the conservative tradition, which has been deeply influenced by religious parties, has given rise to welfare policies that tend to strengthen traditional gender roles within the family. Social rights are associated with employment, and, given the lack of active efforts to bring women into the labor market, they have primarily been provided to men. Women, therefore, enjoy such rights mostly as wives. As mothers, they are given payments through childcare allowances or paid maternity leave, which in turn entrenches their position as caregivers within the house-hold. Strengthening the traditional male-breadwinner family, provision for "atyp-ical" households, such as single mothers, tends to be residual (Esping-Andersen, 1999).

The strategy of relying on the family to provide care services, as expressed by the "male breadwinner model," is a central characteristic of the conservative wel-fare regime in both the continental and the southern European countries (Fraser, 1994; Esping-Andersen, 1999). In this regard the welfare state acts as a supple-mentary force. On the one hand, it extends protection to the wage-earner, on the assumption that he bears sole economic responsibility for the household, which has allowed women to refrain from participating in financially supporting the family and granted them protection as wives and mothers. On the other hand, it provides very few care services outside the family, as reflected by the comparatively small size of the public service sector. Even throughout the 1980s and 1990s, follow-ing the dramatic rise in women's education and the weakening of the single-earner model in Europe, daycare services for infants remained extremely limited. Instead, to compensate for this, certain conservative states (such as Austria, Germany, Italy, France, and Belgium) have begun to provide child-allowances that enable women to stay at home with their infants for the first few years of their lives (Kamerman, 2000; Morgan & Zippel, 2003). In other words, they continue to provide support for women by virtue of their being mothers.

Although countries identified with a conservative welfare regime share com-mon basic characteristics, this regime displays the greatest heterogeneity, both among continental European states (i.e. Misra et al., 2007),[1] and between them

---

[1] For instance, France and Belgium are well known for their provision of care services, as seen in the large supply of daycare centers for babies and young children in comparison to other central

and the southern European countries (e.g. Mingione, 1995; Naldini & Saraceno, 2008; Trifiletti, 1999). Indeed, such is the variety that the three worlds of Esping-Andersen's welfare capitalism (1990) have frequently been extended to four, separating the southern European countries from the continental.

The southern European countries diverge from the typical conservative regime in their "rudimentary welfare state," which relies on a shortage of resources to subsidize social protection and rests on a weaker legal and institutionalized basis (Leibfried, 1992, p. 128). This also translates into less developed family policies, in terms of both financial transfers to families with children and policies that help reconcile family and work. Although most conservative regimes are not employment-supportive, in southern European countries the "familistic model" is more deeply rooted. In general, the more familistic the welfare state, the less generous the family benefits. Thus, social protection and care services in southern European countries are more heavily reliant on the family unit, based on strong solidarity and family interdependency within the nuclear and the extended family (Mingione, 1995; Saraceno, 1994). Moreover, while in countries such as Germany family transfers are often regarded as redundant, given the practice of a family wage (Esping-Andersen, 1999), in Italy, for instance, the traditional family role of the nonworking mothers was not given sufficient protection through additional benefits for the male breadwinner (Trifiletti, 1999). Consequently, in this chapter I have taken two countries to represent the conservative welfare regime: Germany – archetypical of this type of regime – and Italy, a southern European state.

Turning to the gendered outcomes of the male breadwinner model, Figs. 1 and 2 show the comparatively low proportions of working mothers and large number of households with a single male wage-earner that characterize the conservative countries. Italy is the only one of the four countries examined here in which male-breadwinner households are more common than dual-earners. While the overall proportion of women participating in the labor market is low in Italy (less than half of all women of working age), in Germany children constitute the primary obstacle to employment, as shown by the dramatically lower participation rates among women with small children.

The restricted access of women in general and mothers, in particular, to sources of independent income in the conservative countries increases women's dependence on their partners, as illustrated by Fig. 3. Because income from paid employment is the major source of economic autonomy for women, low female participation rates in Germany, and even more so in Italy, are translated into high levels of economic dependency on their husbands' earnings.

However, encouraging employment is not the only way the state can offer financial assistance to women. As mentioned above, tying social rights to motherhood,

---

European countries. It is interesting that this large supply of daycare centers in France and Belgium does not come at the expense of relatively generous financial transfers to mothers who prefer to raise their children at home (but see also Morgan, 2002).

which is more common in this regime, is an alternative way to economically empower women unconditional on their labor market participation. Paid childcare leave – financial support to mothers who choose to raise their children at home for the first few years of their lives – is an example of just that. Sufficient data on paid childcare leave are not available, but further analysis (depicted by the black bar in Fig. 3), which excludes Italy because of missing data, shows that childcare and maternity allowances slightly reduce the dependency levels of German women and bring them into line with the USA, where due to the paucity of these allowances they have almost no effect on the average woman's income. Nonetheless, in contrast to income-related benefits (like parental or maternal leaves), care allowances are on a flat-rate basis and barely reach a third of the average wage, at best (Ferrarini, 2003; OECD, 2005; Morgan & Zippel, 2003). These extremely limited allowances do not provide enough to independently run a household, and as such are only effective when accompanied by the protection of marriage. The fact that such financial support is most common in conservative states and has historically always been low, strengthens the assumption that its aim is not to promote women's economic independence, but rather to strengthen the family institution and its traditional household division of labor.

This assumption is also supported by the widely differing approaches adopted by Italy and Germany regarding single mothers. Table 1 shows that the best protection for women in all countries, but particularly in Italy and Germany, is participation in the labor market. In striking contrast to the low rates of women's employment in Italy and Germany, the rates of single mothers who work are high in both absolute and relative terms. In Italy, the low proportion of single mothers (an indication for the strength of the marital institution), is the main source of protection against poverty for women (see also Casper et al., 1994). Also, both in Italy and Germany, the high percentage of widows and the low percentage of singles shown in the table imply that single parent motherhood in conservative countries is mostly imposed on women rather than a matter of choice. Given the conservative tradition and the lack of employment-supportive policies to reconcile family and work obligations, this is not surprising.

The paucity of care services for infants, which would support women's full-time role as wives and mothers, fits within an economy that traditionally depends on highly committed male labor. In the absence of a large service sector providing women with care services on the one hand and employment on the other, and given the lack of institutional arrangements that have traditionally developed with women's entry into the labor market (such as a supply of part-time jobs), working women in these two countries are expected to integrate within a male economy.

That said, the question of what happens to women who do go out to work is an interesting one. On the one hand, it may be that in societies with a conservative tradition, where religious forces play a central role and further conservative attitudes towards the family in public opinion, women will only enter the labor market when they have no other choice (single mothers, for example). In other words, we might expect the majority of working women to be low-class women whose spouses' earnings are not enough to live off, or single women who do not enjoy the social protection that comes with being married. Alternatively, it may be that women who enter the labor market in such a regime are actually those with a careerist orientation, namely, a relatively selective group of educated women who can compete with men in a labor market that is not adapted to women and does not offer them preferential terms of employment.

Figures 4, 5, 6, and 7 provide some empirical evidence of the second alternative. German women have been fairly successful in attaining positions of power and authority, such as jobs in management. The likelihood that they will reach managerial positions is greater than that of Italian women, and is significantly higher than that of Swedish women. Italian women, who are less successful in reaching positions of power in the labor market, are most successful in maximizing their income. General wage gaps between men and women are substantially lower in Italy, where rates of gender occupational segregation are very small compared with the other countries, and women's penetration into the upper wage quintile is extremely impressive (very nearly reaching equal representation).

Figure 8, which presents labor force participation rates of women from different groups by the two factors that most influence women's employment – motherhood and education – strengthens the concept of selectivity. Whereas in Sweden there are virtually no barriers to employment, that is, all women work regardless of the limitations of motherhood and education, in the other countries this is not the case. In the USA motherhood inhibits employment, but not as severely as in Germany, where motherhood is a major obstacle to entering the labor market, even among educated women. Italy is the most interesting case in this regard: while motherhood is not an obstacle to employment (see also Fig. 1), holding an academic degree is a crucial factor. Nearly all women with a B.A. work – including mothers of preschool children – while nonacademic women show lower rates of employment, even when they do not have children.

Generally speaking, women's achievements in the labor market in Germany and Italy are negatively correlated with their participation rates. If we accept the explanation based on selectivity, then women's achievements in the labor market are a direct outcome of their low rates of participation, as conservatism toward women's employment keeps many women at home – in Germany, mothers to small children, in Italy, the uneducated.

Generally, the findings reveal that Germany and Italy share the same basic pattern of gender stratification, but Italy takes it to the extreme. The measures show that participation levels in Italy are the lowest, and thus the more selective group of women who do work has more impressive access to highly paid positions and enjoys the lowest levels of sex segregation. These findings provide further support of Esping-Andersen's decision to include Germany and Italy under the same welfare regime. Justifying his decision, Esping-Andersen claims (1999, Chapter 5) that the basic principle which lies at the foundation of the conservative welfare state – reliance on the family as the dominant welfare provider – is shared by continental and southern European nations. This shared principle is validated here by its shared outcome – similar patterns of gender stratification.

The Liberal Context – The Dual Model: Equal Opportunities and Class Divisions

In sharp contrast to the conservative regime, in the liberal welfare regime – as in social-democracy – the importance of women's employment as a means for achieving gender equality is widely acknowledged. In the spirit of the liberal tradition, and in the belief that there is no better alternative to the labor market for attaining economic independence, women, like men, are seen as potential earners. However, the conceptions of women as workers and wage earners translate into very different practices in the social-democratic and liberal regimes, despite their common emphasis on paid employment. While the importance of women's employment for attaining gender equality in the social-democratic welfare regime is acknowledged by active state support, in the liberal regime – most notably in the USA – the market is the dominant mechanism for service provision, as well as social protection. Thus, care services that are most relevant to women's employment, such as daycare centers, are mostly bought in the market in accordance with their quality (Morgan, 2005). Likewise, the USA is the only advanced society in which paid maternity leave is not provided universally by the state, but is conditional on private terms of employment (Gornick & Meyers, 2003; Kamerman & Gatenio, 2002; OECD, 2005). The state takes no practical responsibility for the special needs of women as child-bearers and mothers, assuming instead that these are matters of personal responsibility.

The need to work, due to miserly income guarantees, along with incentives to employment in the form of advancing anti-discriminatory legislation and tax credits (Orloff, 2006), results in relatively high rates of women's participation in the labor market, and relatively low economic dependency of women on their spouses, as shown in Figs. 1, 2, and 3. The fact that women in the USA do not enjoy gender-based benefits (such as lengthy maternity leave, or leave to care for sick children), and have to function in the labor market without any concessions, makes them more attractive to employers in the private sector. This is accompanied by a high level of awareness regarding equal opportunities at the workplace and the demand for affirmative action, which helps women compete better with men for prestigious positions. Figures 5 and 6 show that women in the USA, in notable contrast to Swedish women, have succeeded in reaching senior positions in the labor market and are less concentrated in female-type jobs.

It would seem, therefore, that the American dual-earner model has managed to overcome the failures of the two previous regimes – in terms of both getting women into the labor market and affording them access to senior positions. However, the predominance that this regime accords to market forces creates large class differences, which intensify the disadvantages of the more vulnerable and needy groups. This class stratification has two consequences: it deepens wage gaps between men and women on the one hand, and it deepens class differentiation among women on the other. On the one hand, ignoring women's limitations as child-bearers and mothers intensifies their difficulties in competing with men, and increases their chances of being overrepresented at the bottom of the wage hierarchy. The lack of regulation of employment conditions and wages – a central characteristic of the liberal labor market – erodes the wages of the weaker groups, in which women are overrepresented. Indeed, this is held to be the main explanation for the large wage gaps between men and women in liberal markets (Blau & Kahn, 1996, 2003; Mendel & Shalev, 2009), as seen in Fig. 7.

On the other hand, the class stratification characteristic of the American market also creates large class divisions among women themselves (Shalev, 2008). Figure 9 provides empirical evidence for this claim by depicting the wage gaps between high- and low-educated women. As can be seen, the wage gaps between these two groups of women are twice as high in the USA as in any of the other countries. The wide wage gaps among women are an indicator of their diverse abilities to purchase care services in the market. Thus, for many women, the fact that they must attain economic independence without any protective welfare programs beyond those offered by the market comprises a significant disadvantage, critically so for unskilled women. Christopher, England, Smeeding, and Phillips (2002) indicate the poverty risk for different groups in the USA: as groups become weaker and in greater need of state assistance, the chance that they will be poor increases. Thus, women are poorer than men, mothers are poorer than nonmothers, and single mothers are poorest of all. While this is a familiar vulnerability in every society, it is particularly notable in the USA, where poverty rates are much higher than in any other welfare state (Christopher et al., 2002; Table 1).

Figure 8 shows that motherhood still constitutes an obstacle to employment, even among educated women. However, while middle- and upper-class women are protected by their husbands' income, in the USA the lack of support for low-class mothers is a major factor behind the high rates of poverty among women in general, and single mothers in particular. Table 1 shows that nearly all nonworking single mothers in the USA live in poverty, as do nearly half of the working single mothers. These rates are incomparably higher than those of the other countries. Bearing in mind that one quarter of all families in the USA are single-parent families, and that the vast majority of these live in poverty, it would appear that strategies for enhancing gender equality in the liberal regime are of no use to a considerable portion of women.

In conclusion, although advancing women's employment is a common goal for both the liberal and the social-democratic models, the former resembles the conservative model in its reluctance to actively support it. High rates of women's employment in the liberal regime are, therefore, also a result of the lack of protection beyond the market, and, unlike in Sweden, have not succeeded in reducing high levels of poverty among women. A market-oriented welfare state, however, benefits women whose skills enable them to successfully compete with men without assistance from the state. For strong women the liberal labor market provides fertile pasture for success. They do not need the state's help in entering the labor market and are not harmed by the potentially negative consequences of such policies, as in the Swedish case. The maintenance of "gender neutrality," which would seem to justify the lack of benefits to women on the basis of difference, acts in their favor by protecting them from gender-based discrimination and betters their chances of reaching powerful positions in the labor market.

Summary and Conclusions

This study reveals that welfare state strategies, especially the ways in which they encourage or repress women's entry into the labor market, have a crucial bearing on the nature of gender stratification. The different patterns of state intervention succeed in narrowing certain aspects of gender inequality, while widening others. Moreover, the very success of a policy on one count may be a source of its limitation on another, so every welfare regime paints a clear tradeoff. The high levels of gender occupational segregation characteristic of social-democratic labor markets are the result of policies aimed at transferring care-giving work from the family to the labor market via the public sector. Consequently, the more the labor market in social-democratic countries attains its aims – high rates of employment among women and mothers – the more gender-segregated it becomes. In the conservative regime the picture is reversed: based on parameters of occupational segregation and earnings, this traditional society actually has a relatively egalitarian labor market, which is achieved in part by the low levels of women's participation rates. The success of the liberal regime in advancing gender equality also comes at the price of its failures, as the very same state interventions have contradictory consequences for women from different classes.

The attempt made in this chapter to link patterns of gender inequality to modes of state intervention emphasizes the important role of the state. The concept of welfare regimes suggests that each pattern of state intervention, and the configuration of gender stratification which it promotes, operates in a different ideological and political context. As a result, solutions cannot easily be imported from one context to another. Although this does not imply that forward movement is impossible, it does suggest that increased gender equality will entail processes of change that evolve within each specific context. By framing the distinctive patterns of gender stratification across regimes in this chapter, I have highlighted the different challenges that different contexts pose to overcoming gender inequality.

Tables and Figures

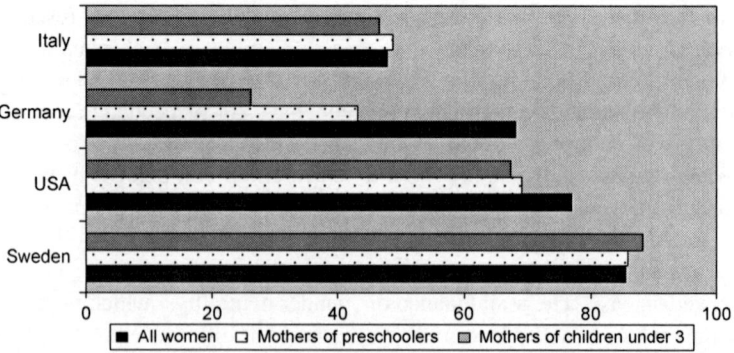

Fig. 1 Labor force participation rates for women (aged 25–60) by motherhood status

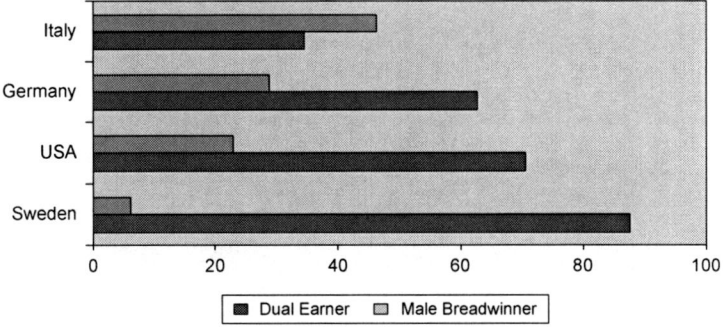

Fig. 2 Distribution of couple-headed households by family type

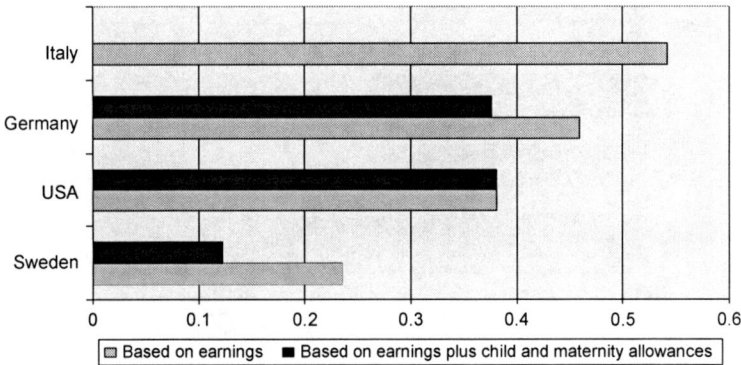

Fig. 3 Women's earnings dependency levels among couple-headed households

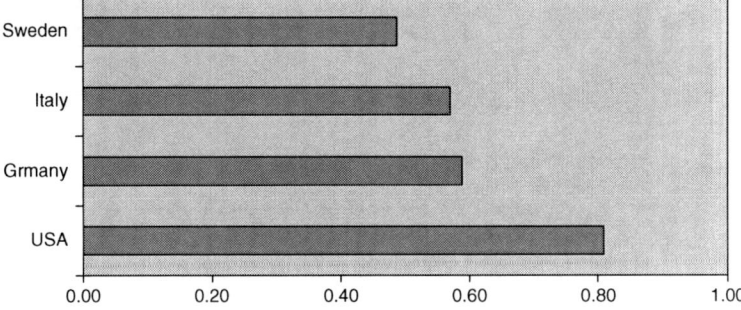

Fig. 4 Gender ratio in managerial positions

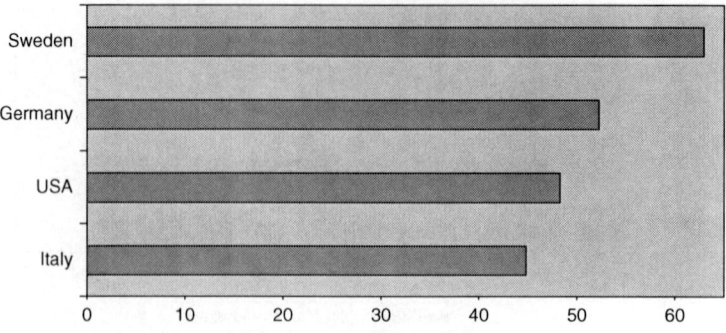

Fig. 5 Occupational sex segregation (index of dissimilarity)

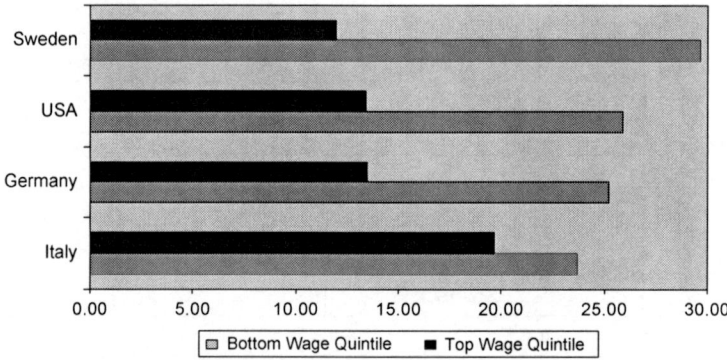

Fig. 6 Women's representation by hourly wage quintile (Note: A value of 20% would imply equal gender representation in a quintile)

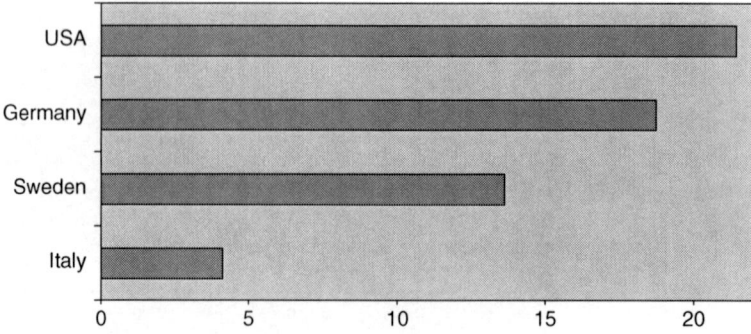

Fig. 7 National gender wage gaps (hourly earnings)

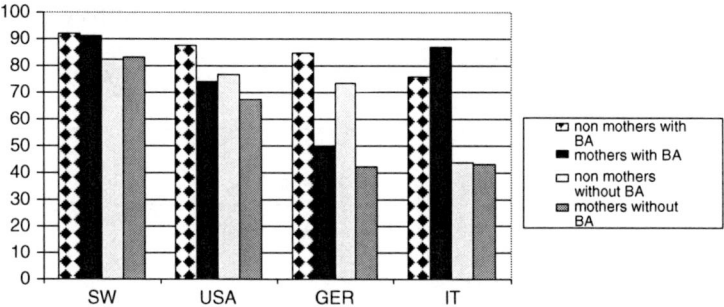

Fig. 8 Labor force participation of women aged 25–60 by education and motherhood

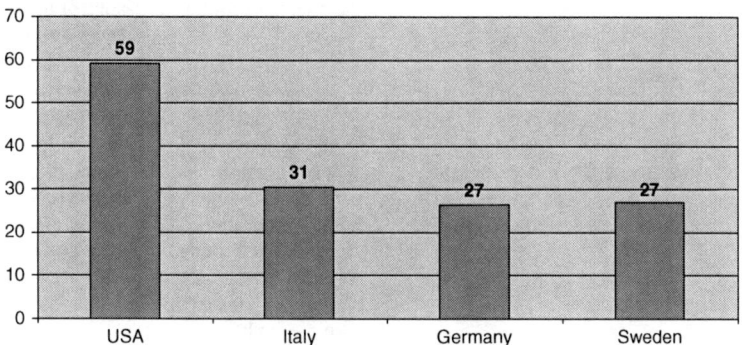

Fig. 9 Wage gaps (%) between women with high and low education

Table 1 Characteristics of single mother families (1990)

	Single mother families (%)	Distribution of single mothers by marital status (%)			Single mothers employed (%)	Employment ratio single mothers/other mothers	Poverty rates[a]	
		Widows	Singles	Divorced or separated			Not in paid work	In paid work
Germany	16	30	23	47	67	1.2	64	11
Italy	5	34	12	54	69	1.7	22	8
Sweden	15	4	46	50	70	0.9	16	4
United States	25	6	35	59	60	0.9	93	43

[a]People in poverty are defined as those whose equivalent disposable income is less than 50% of the average equivalent disposable income in their country.
Source: Kilkey and Bradshaw (1999), Tables 5.1. (pp. 156–157), 5.2 (pp. 158–159), and 5.3 (p. 161).

Appendix 1: Measures and Data Sources of the Gender Inequality Indicators Presented in all figures

Figure No.	Variable	Data source	Definition	Notes
1	Labor force participation	LIS Wave V, except Sweden Wave IV	For women aged 25–60	
2	% Dual-earners households (%) % Male breadwinner (%)	LIS Wave IV	Married or cohabiting couples where both partners have earnings Married or cohabiting couples where only the men have earnings	The figure does not present households with a female sole-breadwinner and those in which none of the spouses have earnings. These households are relatively rare in all countries
3	Women's earning dependency	LIS Wave IV, Except USA Wave V	The gap between the spouses' relative contributions to the household income: Dependency = (male earnings/both spouses' earnings)–(female earnings/both spouses' earnings)	Gray bar: Based on annual earnings Black bar: Based on annual earnings plus child and maternity allowance added to women's earnings
4	Access to managerial positions	All countries LIS; Wave V. Sweden, LNU Survey, 2000	Women (%)/men (%)	
5	Occupational segregation levels	Charles and Grusky (2004, Table 3.3)	Index of dissimilarity (Duncan & Duncan, 1955)	
6	Women's representation by hourly wage quintile	All countries LIS; Wave V. Sweden, LNU Survey, 2000	The proportion of working women in the top and bottom quintiles of their country's earnings distribution	Based on hourly earnings quintiles
7	Gender wage gap	All countries LIS; Wave V. Sweden, LNU Survey, 2000	$100 \times [1 - (\text{average female hourly wage/average male hourly wage})]$	In hourly earnings
8	Labor force participation by motherhood	LIS; All countries Wave V. Sweden Wave IV	Mothers of preschool children (aged 0–6) Nonmothers of preschool children (aged 0–6)	Aged 25–60

Figure No.	Variable	Data source	Definition	Notes
9	Wage gaps between high- and low-educated women	Italy and USA LIS, Wave V. Sweden, LNU, 2000. Germany, GSOEP, 2000	$100 \times [1 - $ (average annual earnings of low-educated/average annual earnings of high-educated)] High and low education was identified according to LIS standardized education levels: low education – up to compulsory education, or initial vocational education. High education – university or college education, or specialized vocational education	

References

Blau, F. D., & Kahn, L. M. (1996). Wage structure and gender earnings differentials – An international comparison. *Economica, 63*(250), 29–62.

Blau, F. D., & Kahn, L. M. (2003). Understanding international differences in the gender pay gap. *Journal of Labor Economics, 21*(1), 106–144.

Bianchi, S. M., Casper, L. M., & Peltola, P. K. (1999). A cross-national look at married women's earnings dependency. *Gender Issues, 17*, 3–33.

Casper, L. M., McLanahan, S. S., & Garfinkel, I. (1994). The gender-poverty gap: What we can learn from other countries. *American Sociological Review, 59*(4), 594–605.

Charles, M., & Grusky, D. B. (2004). *Occupational Ghettos: The Worldwide Segregation of Women and Men*. Stanford, California: Stanford University Press.

Christopher, K. (2002). Welfare state regimes and mothers' poverty. *Social Politics, 9*(1),60–86.

Christopher, K., England, P., Smeeding, T. M., & Phillips, K. R. (2002). The gender gap in poverty in modern nations: Single motherhood, the market, and the state. *Sociological Perspectives, 45*(3), 219–242.

Daly, M. (2000). A fine balance: Women's labor market participation in international comparison. In F. W. Scharpf & V. A. Schmidt (Eds.), *Welfare and work in the open economy* (pp. 467–510). Oxford: Oxford University Press.

Duncan, D., & Duncan, B. (1955). A methodological analysis of segregation indexes. *American Sociological Review, 20*, 210–217.

Ellingsater, A. L. (2009). Leave policy in the Nordic countries: A 'recipe' for high employment/high fertility? *Community, Work and Family, 12*(1), 1–19.

Esping-Andersen, G. (1990). *The three worlds of welfare capitalism*. Cambridge: Polity Press.

Esping-Andersen, G. (1999). *Social foundations of postindustrial economies*. Oxford: Oxford University Press.

Ferrarini, T. (2003). *Parental leave institutions in eighteen post-war welfare states*. Stockholm: Swedish Institute for Social Research Doctoral Dissertation Series No. 58.

Fraser, N. (1994). After the family wage – Gender equity and the welfare state. *Political Theory, 22*(4), 591–618.

Gornick, J. C., & Meyers, M. (2003), *Families that work: Policies for reconciling parenthood and employment*. New York: Russell Sage Foundation.

Gornick, J. C., Meyers, M. K., & Ross, K. E. (1997). Supporting the employment of mothers: Policy variation across fourteen welfare states. *Journal of European Social Policy, 7*(1), 45–70.

Hernes, H. M. (1987). *Welfare state and woman power: Essays in state feminism*. Oslo: Norwegian University Press.

Kamerman, S. B. (2000). *Early childhood education and care (ECEC): An overview of developments in the OECD Countries*. New York: Institute for Child and Family Policy, Columbia University.

Kamerman, S., & Gatenio, S. (2002). *How do America's child benefits compare? Issue brief no. 4*. New York: The Clearinghouse on International Developments in Child, Youth and Family Policies, Columbia University.

Kilkey, M., & Bradshaw, J. (1999). Lone mothers, economic well-being and policies. In D. Sainsbury (Ed.), *Gender and welfare state regimes* (pp. 147–184). Oxford: Oxford University Press.

Korpi, W. (2000). Faces of inequality: Gender, class, and patterns of inequalities in different types of welfare states. *Social Politics, 7*(2), 127–191.

Langan, M., & Ostner, I. (1991). Gender and welfare: Towards a comparative framework. In G. Room (Ed.), *Towards a European welfare state?* (pp. 127–150). Bristol: SAUS.

Leibfried, S. (1992). Towards a European welfare state: On integrating poverty regimes in the European community. In Z. Ferge & J. E. Kolberg (Eds.), *Social policy in a changing Europe* (pp. 245–280). Frankfurt: Campus Verlag.

Lewis, J. (1990). Women's two roles: Myrdal, klein, and post-war feminism. In H. L. Smith (Ed.), *British feminism in the twentieth century* (pp. 167–188). Amherst: University of Massachusetts Press.

Lewis, J. (1992). Gender and the development of welfare regimes. *Journal of European Social Policy, 2*(3), 159–173.

Lewis, J., & Astrom, G. (1992). Equality, difference, and state welfare: Labor market and family policies in Sweden. *Feminist Studies, 18*(1), 59–87.

Mandel, H., & Semyonov, M. (2005). Family policies, wage structures, and gender gaps: Sources of earnings inequality in 20 countries. *American Sociological Review, 70*(6), 949–967.

Mandel, H., & Semyonov, M. (2006). A welfare state paradox: State intervention and women's employment opportunities in 22 countries. *American Journal of Sociology, 111*(6), 1910–1949.

Mandel, H., & Shalev, M. (2009). How welfare states shape the gender pay gap: A theoretical and comparative analysis. *Social Forces, 87*(4), 1873–1911.

Mingione, E. (1995). Labour market segmentation and informal work in Southern Europe. *European Urban and Regional Studies, 2*(2), 121–143.

Misra, J., Budig, M. J., & Moller, S. (2007). Reconciliation policies and the effects of motherhood on employment, earnings and poverty. *Journal of Comparative Policy Analysis, 9*(2), 135–155.

Morgan, K. J. (2002). Does anyone have a "libre choix"? Subversive liberalism and the politics of France's child care policy. In S. Michel & R. Mahon (Eds.), *Child care policy at the crossroads: Gender and welfare state restructuring* (pp. 143–167). New York: Routledge.

Morgan, K. J. (2005). The 'production' of child care: How labor markets shape social policy and vice versa. *Social Politics, 12*(2), 243–263.

Morgan, K. J., & Zippel, K. (2003). Paid to care: The origins and effects of care leave policies in Western Europe. *Social Politics, 10*(1), 49–85.

Naldini, M., & Saraceno, C. (2008). Social and family policies in Italy: Not totally frozen but far from structural reforms. *Social Policy & Administration, 42*(7), 733–748.

O'Connor, J. S. (1993). Gender, class and citizenship in the comparative analysis of welfare state regimes: Theoretical and methodological issues. *The British Journal of Sociology, 44*(3), 501–518.

OECD. (2005). *Can parents afford to work? Childcare costs, tax-benefit policies and work incentives*. Social, Employment and Migration, Working Papers No. 31.

Orloff, A. S. (1993). Gender and the social rights of citizenship – The comparative analysis of gender relations and welfare states. *American Sociological Review, 58*(3), 303–328.

Orloff, A. S. (1996). Gender in the welfare state. *Annual Review of Sociology, 22*, 51–78.

Orloff, A. S. (2006). From maternalism to "employment for all": State policies to promote women's employment across the affluent democracies. In J. D. Levy (Ed.), *The state after statism: New state activities in the age of liberalization* (pp. 230–270). Cambridge, MA: Harvard University Press.

Petersen, T., & Morgan, L. A. (1995). Separate and unequal: Occupation-establishment sex segregation and the gender wage gap. *American Journal of Sociology, 101*(2), 329–365.

Saraceno, C. (1994). The ambivalent familism of the Italian welfare state. *Social Politics, 1*(1), 60–82.

Shalev, M. (2008). Class divisions among women. *Politics & Society, 36*(3), 421–444.

Trifiletti, R. (1999). Southern European welfare regimes and the worsening position of women. *Journal of European Social Policy, 9*(1), 49–64.

Wright, E. O., Baxter, J., & Birkelund, G. E. (1995). The gender gap in workplace authority: A cross-national study. *American Sociological Review, 60*(3), 407–435.

Neighborhoods and Families

James R. McDonell

Introduction

There can be little doubt that neighborhoods and communities[1] play an important role in the lives of the people who live there. The physical and social characteristics of neighborhoods have been associated with health status and morbidity, access to social services, crime and a subjective sense of safety, attainment of education, adolescent risk behavior, child maltreatment, and a host of other well-being indicators (McDonell, 2007; McDonell & Melton, 2008; McDonell & Skosireva, 2009). Indeed, place attachment and the social affiliations that are fostered through a sense of community are central to individual and community well-being (Manzo & Perkins, 2006).

Yet, for many years concern has been growing over the decline of community and the erosion of social connections as a result. More than two decades ago, Putnam (1995) noted a growing tenuousness in the bonds of trust on which people formed social attachments. A decline in social attachment, in turn, reduces the likelihood that local residents will engage in collective action to improve social and economic conditions in their community. Community vitality depends on citizen participation, the absence of which leads to a further erosion of community social life.

There may be good reason to be concerned about the social health of the community and its residents. People are much less engaged with others outside their immediate household than was the case two decades ago (McPherson,

J.R. McDonell (✉)
Institute on Family and Neighborhood Life, Clemson University,
225 S. Pleasantburg Dr., McAlister Square, Suite B11, Greenville, SC 29607, USA
e-mail: jmcdnll@clemson.edu

[1] It is challenging to find terminology that satisfies the variety of ways in which people across the globe refer to residential localities. Neighborhood is, perhaps, the most widely used term, at least in the US, and is generally understood to mean a localized geographic setting consisting of residential and commercial structures that form a relational unit from the perspective of a local resident. This implies that the definition of any one neighborhood may vary from person to person. Neighborhood and community are often used interchangeably to describe areas of varying geography but generally with neighborhood subsumed within community. Other applicable terms include village, hamlet, ward, barrio, and quarter, among others.

M. Ajzenstadt, J. Gal (eds.), *Children, Gender and Families in Mediterranean Welfare States*, Children's Well-Being: Indicators and Research 2, DOI 10.1007/978-90-481-8842-0_3, © Springer Science+Business Media B.V. 2010

Smith-Lovin, & Brashears, 2006). Community residents are less inclined to trust their neighbors and community institutions (Friedman et al., 2007), resulting in declining levels of civic participation, especially among young people (Kelly, 2008). This trend is clearly evident in the results of the annual survey of American college freshmen carried out by the Higher Education Research Institute (Pryor, Hurtado, Saenz, Santos, & Korn, 2007) which showed that students spend less time volunteering and are more distrustful of others, a trend that has been growing with each succeeding cohort of students. Growing distrust means that neighbors are less likely to draw on each other as a source of support, further increasing family social isolation (McDonell, 2009; Melton, 2009).

This rather gloomy view of community social life has been countered by a number of scholars who see a shift in the means through which people maintain social connections. Barman (2005) argued that community engagement has taken a new form in the emergence of social groups that offer alternative pathways for individual membership and novel ways to take collective action. The author cites the emergence of alternative mechanisms, such as charitable giving in the workplace. Kim and Ball-Rokeach 2006 found that connection to an internet-based story-telling network was a significant predictor of neighborhood civic engagement. Other research has also found positive relationships between electronic means of communication and higher levels of community social engagement (Gerodimos, 2008; Hampton & Wellman, 2003).

Whether one sees community as a half-full or half-empty glass, the extent to which social connections among neighbors is waning has enormous implications for child and family well-being. The strains of parenting are eased in the presence of strong social ties (Raikes & Thompson, 2005), especially when children's physical or mental health pose particular challenges (Armstrong, Birnie-Lefcovitch, & Ungar, 2005). At the same time, there is evidence that community characteristics may moderate the effects of social support, leading parents to feel more strain as parents and increasing the likelihood of harsh or punitive parenting (Hill & Herman-Stahl, 2002).

Similarly, children appear to fare well in neighborhoods marked by high levels of social cohesion, where neighbors are more likely to watch out for children and enforce prevailing norms for safety (Nayak, 2003; Sastry & Pebly, 2003). As a result, children feel a greater sense of safety and ease and are better able to use the neighborhood context as a venue for growth and development. Here, too, there is evidence that deleterious neighborhood factors render the community less safe for children, increasing their risk of harm and ill health (McDonell, 2007; McDonell & Skosireva, 2009).

These findings suggest that there is a complex interplay between community characteristics and family and child well-being. Despite increased attention to neighborhood effects among researchers, however, the impact of the community context for children and families is still not well understood. Given this, the purpose of this chapter is to review the state of science with respect to community effects on child and family well-being, drawing implications for policy and research.

Defining Community

Communities are complex, dynamic entities, where currents of change ebb and flow on the tide of human activity. Community boundaries change as jurisdictions of local authority consume newly populated areas nearby. People come and go as opportunity and fortunes rise in some localities and fall in others. Residents grow up, marry, have children, age, and die. Buildings, streets, sidewalks, and parks fall into disrepair and are rebuilt, replaced, or abandoned. Political leaders are swept into power bringing new policy and program priorities to bear, and are then swept out of power to make way for a new round of leaders with new priorities. The community's cultural landscape shifts with the changing attitudes, beliefs, and perceptions of residents and policymakers. It is not surprising, then, that consensus on the definition of community is so elusive.

A logical starting point, however, is to consider community as bounded, physical space. Whether a community's boundaries are determined by law, politics, planning, statistical necessity, convention, affiliation, or a host of other conditions, communities are geographically delimited in ways generally recognizable to the people who live there. Residents are likely to know, at least in a general sense, the borders of their city, town, or village, or what areas are covered by their children's school district and the neighborhood fire district. They may be aware of the area included in their postal code and may know where local transportation hubs are located and the routes that flow out from these locations. These borders, however, are defined by municipal councils, planning boards, or other governmental bodies, often with little, if any, involvement by community residents. These demarcated areas serve the purpose of ordering certain aspects of community life and, as such, relate to residents only in specific ways and at specific times.

To the extent that community residents are concerned about geographic boundaries, it is on a smaller scale. Residents are most likely to identify with and form an attachment to the geographic area most immediate to their dwelling and may come to believe that this sense of place and belonging is shared among their neighbors. Bonds of trust emerge through the shared experience of place and residents learn to rely on each other in an effort to achieve individual and collective goals. The neighborhood becomes increasingly cohesive as residents get to know one another, engage in reciprocal helping, and take collective action to safeguard the community from perceived threats. Residents may form links across geographic neighborhoods through their involvement in civic clubs, faith institutions, and other community groups, strengthening the social fabric of the broader community and providing a network of resources on which to draw in the interests of the local neighborhood.

Community organizations and institutions provide an avenue for residents to take part in the civic life of the broader community of which their neighborhood is a part. This organizational/institutional community is critical to affording local residents a voice in shaping the social, political, and cultural landscape of the community and often serves as a buffer between neighborhood residents and the political and cultural winds that might otherwise batter local residents into acquiescence on matters important to their well-being. It also serves the interests of local government in increasing citizen participation in decision making, seen as an essential guarantee of human rights (Development Research Center on Citizenship, Participation, and Accountability, 2006; Gaventa, 2004).

The neighborhood political community is defined, in part, by the extent to which residents engage local governance structures in efforts to protect the community from outside encroachment (McDonell, 2006). Such actions are influenced by residents' place attachment and perceptions of shared interests, values, and beliefs among neighborhood residents (Best & Strüver, 2000). The vitality of the political community is reflected in residents' beliefs that collective action is an appropriate avenue for bringing about local change, and their willingness to participate in relevant change efforts. Collective efficacy has been shown to be a key element of neighborhood well-being (Duncan & Raudenbush, 2001; Morenoff, Sampson, & Raudenbush, 2001).

Residents are also vital to the vibrancy of the local economy by contributing labor capital and trading in goods and services. Local spending patterns help create and keep jobs in the community. The overall wealth of the community depends on residents making investments through home purchases and upgrades, participating in community financial institutions, paying local taxes, and contributing labor and financial capital to nongovernmental organizations. Community wealth, in turn, is critical to attracting investments, such as new businesses and capital investments in existing businesses, strengthening the local economy and contributing to resident well-being. Children's spending patterns are increasingly recognized as a significant factor in maintaining a strong local economy (National Institute on Media and the Family, 2002).

In summary, community may be defined as a physical place that serves as a context for the complex interplay of social, political, organizational, and economic forces that shape the transactional processes among people and between people and place. These transactions define the core values and ideologies that shape the community normative structure and give life to a collective and cohesive sense of place. The attachments that follow help to sustain the community across time and give it a palpable feeling of contentment and well-being, a sense that the community is a good place to live.

Families in a Global Context

To say that conceptions of family have changed over the last several decades is an understatement. The tide of global change has swept away traditional family forms, leaving new forms in their place. In an era of rapid social and technological change it may be no more valid to talk of families as two adults and their children residing in the same household than to speak of the vast distances separating human settlements on different continents. Families have undergone dramatic and profound changes as the world has become a smaller place. Time will judge the success of law and policy to accommodate the new family reality.

In many parts of the world, single parent families have increased as divorce rates have risen (United Nations Statistics Division, 2008). At the same time, fertility rates have declined in developed countries, falling below replacement rates in some cases, and have increased in some of the least developed states. As a result, families grow smaller in the rich nations and become larger in the poorest parts of the world. While the western democracies implement strategies, such as increasing family allowances and implementing flextime and other family-friendly workplace policies (Government Communication Office, 2009), family size grows instead where family planning services are limited and women feel pressed to reproduce to protect against the loss of children through disease and death, as a result slipping further into economic despair (United Nations Population Fund, 2008; United Nations Conference on Trade and Development, 2008).

Political, economic, and civil strife around the world increasingly displace families from their homes, and many children become separated from their caregivers (Office of the United Nations High Commissioner for Refugees, 2006). The ravages of HIV have orphaned many children, contributing to increases in the number of children living on the street or in institutional settings (Joint United Nations Programme on HIV/AIDS, 2008). It is becoming increasingly common for children to live in households with unrelated caretakers (Green, 2007). In the developing world, children's prospects for the future are significantly dimmed by preventable disease, armed conflict, limited access to education, poverty, and a host of other social ills.

There is growing recognition that the constellation of people comprising a family has changed dramatically and new family forms are increasingly being incorporated in social welfare schemes around the world. For example, the number of countries conferring legal rights on gay and lesbian couples, many of whom are parenting, is growing (Minot, 2003). Single motherhood is more commonplace across socio-economic strata and social welfare schemes supporting single parent families increasingly assure the health and well-being of single mothers and their children (Cunningham-Burley, Backett-Milburn, & Kemmer, 2006; Rowlingson & McKay, 2006).

Evidence suggests that cohabitation, couples living together without marriage, has become a typical life-course experience, with many couples either cohabiting as a means of testing compatibility prior to marriage or choosing to remain together as an unmarried couple. Cohabiting couples tend to delay having children and have fewer children, contributing to declining birth rates in countries with high rates of cohabitation (Popenoe, 2008). Whether due to cohabitation or other reasons, many women are choosing to delay childbearing, giving them the opportunity to make a successful transition to adulthood before taking on the demands of motherhood, and thus increasing well-being outcomes for their children (National Research Council, 2005).

Finally, a substantial number of adult children are returning to live with their parents after having established households of their own. The reasons for doing so vary, but include the need to care for aging parents, financial barriers to living on one's own, the health or physical disability of the returning child, among others (Beaupré,

Turcotte, & Milan, 2008). The co-residence of adult children and their parents does not necessarily lead to tensions in the home, although frustrations do arise. Rather, aging parents may find it rewarding to have someone to assist with household chores and contribute financially to maintaining the household. At the same time, children may find that living with adult parents reduces expenses, allowing children to save to meet life goals (Turcotte, 2006; Velkoff, 2002).

Clearly, the changing global economic, political, and social context has affected families in ways that are only now beginning to be understood. How these transitions are likely to affect children and families over the long term remains to be seen. Some states are beginning to respond by adopting policies and programs responsive to changing family needs, recognizing that fundamental human rights issues are at stake. Other states struggle to maintain traditional family forms, doggedly refusing to accept that change is in the wind and cloaking religious morality in the garb of political debate. In the long run, such a view is detrimental to the general social well-being.

Community Effects on Families and Children

Despite several decades of research, surprisingly little is known about community effects on family well-being, although substantial progress is evident. There are several factors accounting for this. The complex, bi-directional nature of the relationships between people and place makes it difficult to capture much variability, reducing statistical models to data on a few easily obtainable factors. This is compounded by the lack of standard definitions for community, limiting comparisons across studies as researchers idiosyncratically construct units of analyses. The complexity of community also poses challenges in finding adequate comparisons for effects models. Finally, the development of measures and measurement strategies has not kept pace with theory, and the over-reliance on single source measures, typically surveys or macro-level data, does little to clear up the noise in statistical models (Coulton, Korbin, Chan, & Su, 2001; McDonell, 2006).

The picture today is much clearer than ever before as increased attention is given to small area indicators of family and child well-being and as the technologies of community effects research improve. As a result, the range of indicators and outcomes being examined through a community lens has broadened considerably. In a limited space it is not feasible to adequately cover the range of the research on community effects on children and families. Therefore, this chapter focuses on selected issues within the broader topics of parenting, health, safety, achievement, and general well-being.

Effects on Parenting

Less than a decade ago, the view in the scientific community was that community characteristics had little effect on parenting and that variability in family management practices could be attributed to family characteristics more than to the context in which parenting occurred (National Research Council and Institute of Medicine, 2000). In part, this reflects the fact that much of the available research focused on parenting as a mediator of children's exposure to egregious community social conditions rather than on parent–child interactions and tended to rely on macro-level indicators of community effects (McDonell, 2007). Macro-structural factors, such as poverty and crime rates, may indicate the general character of a community but often do so too broadly to say much about the lives of the people who live there.

Recent research, however, more clearly demonstrates the effects of community characteristics on parenting, showing that contextual factors explain a good deal more of the differences in parenting than was once believed. In a review of the literature, Kotchick and Forehand (2002) found evidence that the social and physical characteristics of communities had an effect on the decisions parents make regarding how much freedom children are allowed and the type and range of activities in which they are permitted to participate. Similarly, Beyers, Bates, and Dodge (2003) found that less parental monitoring was associated with children's problematic community behavior. However, this was moderated by the stability of the neighborhood, suggesting greater neighborhood cohesion and an increased likelihood of neighbor-to-neighbor support.

Neighborhood characteristics have been found to affect the strategies parents use to keep children safe from harm. For example, Letiecq and Koblinsky (2004) found that African-American fathers were more likely to monitor children closely, teach children about neighborhood risks, and take direct action to protect children when they perceived the neighborhood to be dangerous. Kling, Liebman, and Katz (2001) suggested that the pervasive atmosphere of fear in dangerous neighborhoods led mothers to isolate themselves and to monitor children's activities more closely. An intense focus on children and greater restrictions on children's autonomy is likely to increase family tensions and reduce parental nurturing. Less parental nurturing and decreased family cohesion has the paradoxical effect of increasing children's exposure to violence and other community dangers (Gorman-Smith, Henry, & Tolan, 2004).

Parenting is generally less stressful when parents perceive that social support is available, whether or not such support is utilized. However, research has shown that community characteristics moderate the buffering effect of social support, potentially leading to more restrictive and punitive parenting practices. The unpredictable nature of distressed communities may lead parents to place more restrictions on children's outdoor activity. This reduces opportunities for social support, contributing to family social isolation, and increasing family stress (Hill & Herman-Stahl, 2002). Ceballo and McLoyd (2002) found that parental nurturing decreased as neighborhood quality declined, even in the presence of social support.

There is evidence that the cohesiveness of the community has an effect on parenting practices. Silk, Sessa, Morris, Steinberg, and Avenevoli (2004) found that the effects of a hostile parenting style on children were less severe when children perceived the community to be cohesive. This suggests that children make use of adult support in the neighborhood to offset the tumultuousness of home life. Soubhi, Raina, and Kohen (2004) found that children were less likely to be at risk of injury in cohesive neighborhoods, even when parenting practices, such as low levels of parental supervision, indicated a greater risk of harm for children. Finally, McDonell (2007) found that parents were more nurturing of their children in neighborhoods marked by indications of resident watchfulness. Presumably, neighborhood vigilance indicates more cohesive neighborhoods where parents feel assured that someone is watching out for their children.

Effects on Health

Community characteristics have been found to exert considerable influence over the health of residents. Cohen et al. (2003) found that neighborhood physical deterioration, as indicated by the presence of abandoned and boarded-up dwellings, was associated with increased mortality from all causes and the morbidity of sexually transmitted diseases. The authors posed the possibility that neighborhood physical condition had an adverse impact on healthy behavior within social networks. Ellen, Mijanovich, and Dillman (2001) proposed two causal pathways for neighborhood effects on resident health status. First, neighborhoods influence attitudes and behaviors over the short-term, affecting health outcomes susceptible to proximal neighborhood conditions. Second, the stresses associated with neighborhood distress over time wears down residents' resistance, making them more susceptible to long-term health consequences.

Debrand and colleagues (2008) found that living in a neighborhood characterized by low levels of resident mobility, that is, where residents had few opportunities to move from one community to another in the interest of economic or social opportunities, was associated with poor self-reported health outcomes. However, Bures (2003) found that a retrospective assessment of residential stability in childhood was associated with higher self-assessments of global health at midlife. These contradictory findings may reflect neighborhood economic conditions, which, on the one hand, trapped residents in a poor neighborhood by limiting the financial resources to migrate to another community in search of a better life and, on the other hand, controlled for neighborhood economic status.

Sastry and Pebley (2003) found significant but modest neighborhood effects on children's health in a large-scale study of families and neighborhoods in Los Angeles. Neighborhood factors included median household income, neighborhood-level concentration of immigrants, and residential stability. The combined neighborhood effects were significant for general health status, as reported by an adult caregiver, and for specific health conditions including chronic conditions, ear infections, asthma, obesity, and anemia. The only health outcome not significantly related to neighborhood conditions was whether or not the child had ever been hospitalized. The study suggests the pervasiveness of community effects on health status.

Wen and Zhang (2007) assessed the effects of neighborhood conditions on residents' propensity to exercise. While there was a good deal of variability between neighborhoods, the study found that neighborhood deprivation reduced the odds of community residents reporting having exercised at any time over the past year while social capital, the presence of restaurants and bars, and the presence of community arts and cultural facilities increased the odds in specific neighborhoods. Aggregate education increased the odds of residents reporting having exercised at least once per week while block density lowered the odds. Finally, mixed land use substantially increased the odds of residents reporting having exercised at least four times per week.

Laraia, Messer, Evenson, and Kaufman (2007) assessed the effects of neighborhood characteristics on physical activity during pregnancy. The authors found that higher levels of physical incivilities, such as the presence of graffiti and housing deterioration, was associated with decreased odds of physical activity before pregnancy and decreased odds of weight gain during pregnancy. In addition, the level of neighborhood social activity, indicated by such factors as parks, sidewalks, porches, and the presence of people on the street, was directly associated with the odds of inadequate and excessive weight gain. These findings support the general body of research showing the importance of neighborhood physical and social characteristics for physical activity and health-related outcomes.

Effects on Safety

Researchers have identified a number of community factors that impact resident safety and perceptions of safety, with much of the research focused on children. For example, Zani, Cicognani, and Albanesi (2001) found that adolescents in large urban environments felt less safe and less attached to the community than did adolescents in moderately sized urban environments and small towns. Adolescents in smaller towns reported feeling a much greater sense of social connection than did adolescents in larger communities. Kirk and Gannon-Rowley (2003) found that collective efficacy and neighborhood social disorder differentiated students' sense of safety across schools and communities. However, the variability in subjective safety was greater across students within schools than it was across schools and communities.

Beh-Arieh, McDonell, and Attar-Schwartz (2009) found that teachers generally felt that children were safer before and after school and on the way to and from school than did the children themselves. Parents' showed much greater concern for children's safety at and en route to school than did either children or teachers. The authors concluded that the difference in sense of safety between students and teachers reflects the fact that children are more likely to experience incidents suggesting a lack of safety at higher rates than are teachers. Parents concerns about safety may well reflect their limited awareness of what transpires in children's lives at school and in the immediate environment of the school. This is supported by Austin, Furr, and Spine (2002) who found that quality of neighborhood housing had a positive effect on neighborhood satisfaction and perceptions of safety among residents, except among residents who had been victimized. In the latter case this resulted in a negative effect on neighborhood satisfaction and perceptions of safety.

Reading, Haynes, and Shenassa (2005) found that high poverty rates and poor quality of housing was associated with an increased risk of child injuries, independent of risks associated with family characteristics. The authors noted, however, that poverty and material deprivation are necessary but insufficient indicators of child injury risk. That is, injury risk is lower in some neighborhoods that are highly distressed while being much higher in neighborhoods that are less distressed. This suggests that additional research is needed to identify other factors implicated in children's risk of injuries.

A study by McDonell and Skosireva (2009) is suggestive in this regard. The study examined the effect of community characteristics measured through an observational rating scale to predict children's injuries at the neighborhood level as indicated by geocoded rates of ICD-9-CM[2] coded hospital discharge diagnoses. Neighborhood characteristics included indicators of neighborhood physical and social appearance, social engagement, barrier density, safety, and amenities. The overall model was significant and accounted for 46.0% of the variance in rates of injuries per 1,000 children, with neighborhood physical appearance contributing the most to the explained variance.

Children are at a greater risk of injury in neighborhoods marked by high levels of social and economic distress. However, a number of factors mediate such risk. Soubhi et al. (2004) found that neighborhood cohesion attenuates the risk of injury to children even in the presence of neighborhood problems and families' low-income status that otherwise significantly predict children's injuries. Tester, Rutherford, Wald, and Rutherford (2004) found that children who lived within a block of a speed bump were significantly less likely to sustain a roadway injury than were children who lived in neighborhoods where traffic speeds were not controlled by such barriers.

In a related vein, Schieber and Vegega (2002) noted that innovations in community infrastructure design may place children at risk of roadway injuries. The trend toward wider roads to accommodate large tractor trailers may make street crossings too wide for children to cross safely during a light change. Wider roadways also eliminate sidewalks, wide shoulders, and refuge islands, increasing the risk that children may be injured while crossing a street. This is especially a risk to children who walk to school and who may not always be as attentive as necessary to road traffic.

Finally, there is growing research on how neighborhood effects relate to child maltreatment. Coulton, Crampton, Irwin, Spilsbury, and Korbin (2007) reviewed the literature to identify the links between neighborhood characteristics and child maltreatment, finding strong connections between neighborhood structural factors, especially neighborhood economic conditions, and child maltreatment. The authors

---

[2] The United States has yet to adopt later versions of the International Classification of Diseases (ICD) that are in general use elsewhere in the world, and still relies on the clinical modification of the 9th version of the ICD.

also linked neighborhood processes, such as reciprocal helping and social support, neighboring, and other social engagement factors, and child maltreatment, although these effects were generally weaker than those of neighborhood structural characteristics.

McDonell (2007) looked at the connection between neighborhood characteristics and residents' perceptions of the extent to which a neighbor with a young child takes steps to assure children's safety at home. Such actions as using safety gates, restraining children in the car, putting caps on electrical outlets and the like may indicate the general extent to which young children's safety needs are being neglected, potentially indicating child neglect more broadly. The study found that such factors as neighborhood physical appearance, the condition of parks and public spaces, the density of residential symbols signaling neighbors to stay away, and the adequacy of rubbish bins significantly predicted the extent to which children's safety in the home was assured, accounting for 23% of the variance in measures of safety.

Effects on Achievement

Community characteristics have been found to significantly affect children's achievement. For example, Biddulph, Biddulph, and Biddulph (2003) identified a number of community factors affecting achievement among Maori children in New Zealand. Social networks were critical to helping families maintain cultural ties and were important sources of support as parents sought to improve their children's achievement outcomes. Peer groups may have a positive effect by reinforcing children's achievement goals but may have a negative effect to the extent that peer group influences override parental expectations. Access to community resources, including community centers, libraries, health care providers, and social care providers enhance children's achievement far beyond what schools alone are able to do. Finally, prevailing community norms concerning gender may strengthen gender identity as it relates to achievement expectations but may also result in children avoiding opportunities they feel may label them with unflattering gender stereotypes.

Plybon, Edwards, Butler, Belgrave, and Allison (2003) found that perceptions of higher neighborhood cohesion were associated with higher levels of educational self-efficacy and grades among African-American adolescent girls, controlling for maternal education. Further, increased use of social support as a coping strategy was also positively associated with educational self-efficacy. However, a study by Kauppinen (2007) found no neighborhood effects on rates of educational attainment among residents of Helsinki. On the other hand, in this case, neighborhood characteristics did influence the type of education completed (upper secondary versus vocational school).

Nash (2002) found that students' sense of school coherence, the extent to which the school experience was perceived to be meaningful, manageable, and comprehensible, mediated the effects of neighborhood social control and a negative peer culture on students' educational behavior, reducing students' risk of school failure. This suggests the importance of the school environment for children, offsetting the deleterious effects of other neighborhood conditions.

Harding (2003) found that of two groups of children matched on family characteristics that experience different levels of neighborhood economic distress during adolescence, the group in the more economically distressed neighborhood was at greater risk of school drop-out than was the group in the less distressed neighborhood.

Ainsworth (2002) found that collective socialization, social capital, social control, perceived opportunity, and institutional characteristics mediated neighborhood effects on children's educational outcomes, and accounted for about 40% of the variance in neighborhood effects on educational attainment. This suggests that neighborhood social processes are important factors in children's educational outcomes, and may have greater potency than do neighborhood physical characteristics.

Finally, Leventhal and Brooks-Gunn (2004) found that moving to a low poverty neighborhood had a positive effect on the academic achievement of male teenagers compared to those males who remained in high poverty neighborhoods. Further, males in the low poverty neighborhoods had test scores comparable to females in the same neighborhood while males in high poverty neighborhoods scored 10 points lower on average than females in the same neighborhood. These results show that neighborhood economic distress alone has a significant effect on how well children perform in school.

Effects on General Well-Being

Neighborhood effects research has examined a range of other outcomes, although not to the extent of those discussed above. For example, Widome, Sieving, Harpin, and Hearst (2008) found that adolescents who expressed low intentions to contribute to neighborhood improvement and who indicated limited familiarity with neighbors and neighborhood support opportunities reported higher levels of involvement in violence than did young people who were more connected to their neighborhood. On a related dimension, Wilcox, Quisenberry, and Jones (2003) found that higher rates of businesses, parks, and playgrounds increased residents' perceptions of community danger but that these effects were attenuated when controlling for crime rates.

There is evidence that the social climate of the neighborhood is related to the community behavior of young children. Caughy, O'Campo, and Nettles (2008) found, for example, that children who lived in neighborhoods marked by high degrees of social disorder and fear of crime and violence were significantly more likely to be anxious and depressed than were children who lived in less disordered neighborhoods. The authors also found that children had fewer behavior problems when there were greater opportunities for children to become involved in the community. Other studies have found that civic engagement is associated with fewer community social problems (Bowen, Gwisada, & Brown, 2004; Family Strengthening Policy Center, 2005; Scott, Taylor, & Blakester, 2005).

Interestingly, a study by Grogan-Kaylor and Otis (2007) found that community characteristics did not predict parents' use of corporal punishment. This seems to contradict other findings that neighborhood characteristics, especially disorder and fear of crime, were positively associated with harsh or punitive parenting strategies. It is likely that this finding is a result of the generality of community factors used as predictors. For the most part, this consisted of regional variation and economic measures of neighborhood quality. These factors are far too broad and remote from the actual neighborhood context to be predictive of much of anything at the local level.

Finally, Shinn and Toohey (2003) suggested that many observers tend to under-estimate the effects of context on human behavior. In a review of the literature, the authors identified a number of dimensions of community deemed critical to understanding community effects. These included social disorder, the normative environment, and collective efficacy, which were among the factors that emerged from research carried out in urban neighborhoods in Chicago (cf. Sampson, 2003; Sampson, Morenoff, & Earls, 1999). Other identified factors were social stress and incivilities, which reflect the extent of physical decline in neighborhoods, and resources, social capital, and sense of community, factors reflecting the basis on which resident collective action for change may be built.

Conclusions

This brief review of the relationship between community characteristics and fami-lies amply demonstrates the powerful impact of place on people's lives. However, the picture is much more complex than is explicated here. The interactions between community factors at the macro-level, such as community economic distress or the distribution of demographic factors, and those at the micro-level, including features of community design or the observable quality of housing stock and resident social engagement, makes the task of sorting out community effects all the more chal-lenging. Add individual characteristics, family structural characteristics, and social processes to the mix and the task becomes exponentially more difficult. It should not be surprising to see community effects researchers babbling incoherently in the dark recesses of their data files.

Still, considerable progress has been made, clearing up the picture just enough to motivate researchers to press on. Better measurement tools and more powerful and sophisticated analytic strategies help bring a broader range of community effects into the research fold. The volume of studies is increasing as the preponderance, subtlety, and quality of the research attracts new researchers to the field. Still, there are many gaps in what is known about neighborhood effects and a lack of consensus among researchers on how the unit of analysis is defined and the most efficacious approaches to the design of community effects research.

A new understanding, that the community physical and social context has far more to do with the course of peoples' lives than was once believed, is beginning to emerge in the field. Research studies are sorting out which community factors have a direct effect on residents, where these effects are mediated by individual, family, and community factors, where and when these effects occur, and at what level of magnitude the effects occur. We have not reached the pinnacle of understanding by any stretch of the imagination and there are times when it seems the journey is a maddening confusion of misdirection and dead ends. Out of these fits and starts, however, a fairly good road map is emerging. Researchers are not as lost as might be believed.

Unfortunately, the emerging portrait of community effects is not being translated into policy and program action as quickly as it might be. Perhaps social scientists are just not very good at getting information into the hands of people who might use it to bring about change in peoples' lives. Perhaps policy makers and program planners do not know how to translate information at their disposal into action. Or it may well be that the actions taken are influenced more by political and economic considerations than by information suggesting otherwise. A case in point in this regard is found in research showing that community design features, such as wider roadways to accommodate larger trucks, places people at risk of injury while crossing the street. Apparently, the economics of transporting goods through or near residential communities outweighs the science.

Many of the community factors reviewed in this chapter are amenable to change. Traffic in neighborhoods may be slowed by adding speed bumps, lowering speed limits while increasing enforcement, installing signs indicating children at play in the neighborhood, and other low-cost alternatives. Including L- or T-shaped intersections in new housing developments, and eliminating or modifying through streets in residential neighborhoods will also slow traffic and reduce property theft and other crimes of opportunity.

Taking steps to improve the social organization of residential areas, such as fostering neighborhood associations, neighborhood watch groups, and the like is an effective strategy for increasing community engagement and resident-to-resident social engagement. Existing community organizations and institutions may be willing to create opportunities for resident social engagement. An anecdotal example is that of a small suburban fire department that began planning and implementing family support activities, such as financial education and parenting groups, at the fire station. This effort was so successful that when a new fire house was built, the fire department added a front porch, complete with rocking chairs in adult and child sizes, and a room for a small family support center. The fire house has become a hub of community activities.

Community beautification projects are also relatively inexpensive. Assuring that adequate public trash bins are available and regularly emptied, organizing community clean-up campaigns, getting local volunteers to repair dwellings for residents who cannot afford to spruce up their homes, planting flowers and shrubbery in public spaces, forming community garden projects, and related activities are an effective means of reducing community incivilities. Residents will begin to take greater pride in the neighborhood and will be more likely to engage their neighbors in maintaining an improved community appearance.

Engaging community residents in the planning process especially with respect to policy decisions which ultimately have a direct bearing on the lives of community residents is an effective strategy for strengthening civic engagement. This practice has the added benefit of giving policy makers the perspective of community residents when planning for the community. To be truly effective, however, this must go beyond holding public hearings and soliciting resident reactions to proposed policy initiatives. Rather, it must include substantive mechanisms for residents to have a voice in the planning process. The process must be a partnership between policy makers and community residents in which residents have a real opportunity to shape policy decisions.

Taking actions such as those noted above go a long way to creating cohesive communities. Cohesive communities are far more likely to take steps to protect the community, safeguard the safety of community residents, and foster neighbor-to-neighbor social interaction and support. In turn, residents will show a greater propensity to join together in common cause to improve community conditions in ways that benefit all those who live there. The normative structure of the community will be strengthened in ways that reflect the goals of the community as a whole and the individual families residing there. This is the hallmark of a healthy community.

The overarching challenge, however, is in getting policy makers to pay greater attention to community factors in community planning. The physical and social features of community are frequently overlooked in policy development or are overshadowed by political interests. Social service providers do not often consider the context of the lives of the people they serve and may well seek to bring about change in people rather than changes in the community as a way of redressing social ills. Thus, focus must be put on devising more effective strategies for bringing community effects to the fore and assuring that the right information is getting into the right hands at the right time.

References

Ainsworth, J. (2002). Why does it take a village? The mediation of neighborhood effects on educational achievement. *Social Forces, 81*(1), 117–152.

Armstrong, M. I., Birnie-Lefcovitch, S., & Ungar, M. T. (2005). Pathways between social support, family well-being, quality of parenting, and child resilience: What we know. *Journal of Child and Family Studies, 14*(2), 269–281.

Austin, D., Furr, A., & Spine, M. (2002). The effects of neighborhood conditions on perceptions of safety. *Journal of Criminal Justice, 30*, 417–427.

Barman, E. (2005, August 12). *Of place and purpose: Competing visions of community in the non-profit sector.* Paper presented at the annual meeting of the American Sociological Association, Philadelphia, PA.

Beaupré, P., Turcotte, P., & Milan, A. (2008, November 21). *Junior comes back home: Trends and predictors of returning to the parental home.* Retrieved from http://www.statcan.gc.ca/pub/11-008-x/2006003/pdf/9480-eng.pdf

Beh-Arieh, A., McDonell, J., & Attar-Schwartz, S. (2009). Safety and home-school relations as indicators of children's well-being: Whose perspective counts? *Social Indicators Research, 90*, 339–349.

Best, U., & Strüver, A. (2000). *The politics of place: Critical of spatial identities and critical spatial identities*. Tokyo: International Critical Geography Group.

Beyers, J., Bates, J. P., & Dodge, K. (2003). Neighborhood structure, parenting processes, and the development of youth's externalizing behaviors: A multi-level analysis. *American Journal of Community Psychology, 31*(1/2), 35–53.

Biddulph, F., Biddulph, J., & Biddulph, C. (2003). *The complexity of community and family influences on children's achievement in New Zealand: Best evidence synthesis*. Wellington: Ministry of Education.

Bowen, L., Gwisada, V., & Brown, M. (2004). Engaging community residents to prevent violence. *Journal of Interpersonal Violence, 19*, 356–367.

Bures, R. (2003). Childhood residential stability and health at midlife. *American Journal of Public Health, 93*(7), 1144–1148.

Caughy, M. O., O'Campo, P. J., & Nettles, S. M. (2008). The effect of residential neighborhood on child behavior problems in first grade. *American Journal of Community Psychology, 42*(1–2), 39–50.

Ceballo, R., & McLoyd, V. (2002). Social support and parenting in poor dangerous neighborhoods. *Child Development, 73*, 1310–1321.

Cohen, D., Mason, K., Bedimo, A., Scribner, R., Basolo, V., & Farley, T. (2003). Neighborhood physical conditions and health. *American Journal of Public Health, 93*(3), 467–471.

Coulton, C., Crampton, D., Irwin, M., Spilsbury, J., & Korbin, J. (2007). How neighborhoods influence child maltreatment: A review of the literature and alternative pathways. *Child Abuse & Neglect, 31*, 1117–1142.

Coulton, C. J., Korbin, J., Chan, T., & Su, M. (2001). Mapping residents' perceptions of neighborhood boundaries: A methodological note. *American Journal of Community Psychology, 29*(2), 371–383.

Cunningham-Burley, S., Backett-Milburn, K., & Kemmer, D. (2006). Constructing health and sickness in the context of motherhood and paid work. *Sociology of Health & Illness, 28*(4), 385–409.

Debrand, T., Pierre, A., Allonier, C., & Lucas, V. (2008). *Health status, neighborhood effects, and public choice: Evidence from France*. Paris: Institut de recherche et documentation en économie de la santé.

Development Research Centre on Citizenship, Participation, and Accountability. (2006). *Building effective states: Taking a citizen's perspective*. Sussex, UK: Development Research Centre on Citizenship, Participation, and Accountability.

Duncan, G. J., & Raudenbush, S. W. (2001). Neighborhoods and adolescent development: How can we determine the links? In A. Booth & A. C. Crouter (Eds.), *Does it take a village? Community effects on children, adolescents, and families* (pp. 105–136). State College, PA: Pennsylvania State University Press.

Ellen, I., Mijanovich, T., & Dillman, K.-N. (2001). Neighborhood effects on health: Exploring the links and assessing the evidence. *Journal of Urban Affairs, 23*(3–4), 391–408.

Family Strengthening Policy Center. (2005). *Community violence prevention as a family strengthening strategy*. Retrieved from http://www.nasembly.org/fspc/practce/documents/vpdraft_2.pdf

Friedman, S. R., Mateu-Gelabert, P., Curtis, R., Maslow, C., Bolyard, M., Sandoval, M., et al. (2007). Social capital or networks, negotiations and norms? A neighborhood case study. *American Journal of Preventive Medicine, 32*(6 Suppl.), s160–s170.

Gaventa, J. (2004). Strengthening participatory approaches to local governance: Learning the lessons from abroad. *National Civic Review, 93*(4), 16–27.

Gerodimos, R. (2008). Mobilising young citizens in the UK: A content analysis of youth and issue websites. *Information, Communication & Society, 11*(7), 964–988.

Gorman-Smith, D., Henry, D., & Tolan, P. (2004). Exposure to community violence and violence perpetration: The protective effects of family functioning. *Journal of Clinical Child and Adolescent Psychology, 33*(3), 439–449.

Green, M. (2007). *Background paper for Global Partners' Forum: Background paper for high level meeting on children affected by HIV/AIDS*. New York: UNICEF.

Grogan-Kaylor, A., & Otis, M. (2007). The predictors of parental use of corporal punishment. *Family Relations, 56*, 80–91.

Hampton, K., & Wellman, B. (2003). Neighboring in Netville: How the Internet supports community and social capital in a wired suburb. *City & Community, 2*(4), 277–311

Harding, D. (2003). Counterfactual models of neighborhood effects: The effect of neighborhood poverty on dropping out and teenage pregnancy. *American Journal of Sociology, 109*(3), 679–719.

Hill, N. E., & Herman-Stahl, M. A. (2002). Neighborhood safety and social involvement: Associations with parenting behaviors and depressive symptoms among African-American and Euro-American mothers. *Journal of Family Psychology, 16*, 209–219.

Joint United Nations Programme on HIV/AIDS. (2008). *Report on the global HIV/AIDS epidemic 2008*. Geneva: UNAIDS.

Kauppinen, T. (2007). Neighborhood effects in a European city: Secondary education of young people in Helsinki. *Social Science Research, 36*(1), 421–444.

Kelly, D. C. (2009). In preparation for adulthood: Exploring civic participation and social trust among young minorities. *Youth & Society, 40*, 526–540.

Kim, Y. C., & Ball-Rokeach, S. J. (2006). Neighborhood storytelling resources and civic engagement: A multi-level approach. *Human Communication Research, 32*(4), 411–439.

Kirk, D., & Gannon-Rowley, T. (2003, August 16). *Contextual effects on students' safety: Modeling differential effects of neighborhood and school social organization*. Retrieved from http://www.allacademic.com/meta/p107337_index.html

Kling, J. R., Liebman, J. B., & Katz, L. F. (2001). Bullets don't got no name: Consequences of fear in the ghetto. In T. S. Weisner (Ed.), *Discovering successful pathways in children's development: Mixed methods in the study of childhood and family life* (pp. 243–282). Chicago: University of Chicago Press.

Kotchick, B., & Forehand, R. (2002). Putting parenting in perspective: A discussion of the contextual factors that shape parenting practices. *Journal of Child and Family Studies, 11*, 255–269.

Laraia, B., Messer, L., Evenson, K., & Kaufman, J. S. (2007). Neighborhood factors associated with physical activity and adequacy of weight gain during pregnancy. *Journal of Urban Health, 84*(6), 793–806.

Letiecq, B., & Koblinsky, S. (2004). Parenting in violent neighborhoods: African-American fathers share strategies for keeping kids safe. *Journal of Family Issues, 25*, 715–734.

Leventhal, T., & Brooks-Gunn, J. (2004). A randomized study of neighborhood effects on low-income children's educational outcomes. *Developmental Psychology, 40*(4), 488–507.

Manzo, L. C., & Perkins, D. D. (2006). Finding common ground: The importance of place attachment to community participation and planning. *Journal of Planning Literature, 20*(4), 335–350.

McDonell, J. (2006). Indicator measurement in comprehensive community initiatives. In A. Ben-Arie & R. George (Eds.), *Indicators of children's well-being: Understanding their role, usage, and policy influence* (pp. 33–43). Dordrecht, Netherlands: Springer-Verlag.

McDonell, J. (2009). *Strong communities neighborhood survey*. Unpublished raw data.

McDonell, J. R. (2007). Neighborhood characteristics, parenting, and children's safety. *Social Indicators Research, 83*, 177–179.

McDonell, J. R., & Melton, G. B. (2008). Toward a science of community intervention. *Family & Community Health, 31*(2), 113–125.

McDonell, J. R., & Skosireva, A. (2009). Neighborhood characteristics, child injuries, and child maltreatment. *Child Indicators Research, 2*(2), 133–153.

McPherson, M., Smith-Lovin, L., & Brashears, M. E. (2006). Social isolation in America: Changes in core discussion networks over two decades. *American Sociological Review, 71*, 353–375.

Melton, G. B. (2009). How Strong Communities restored my faith in humanity: Children can live in safety. In K. Dodge & D. Coleman (Eds.), *Community-based treatment of child maltreatment* (pp. 82–101). New York: Guilford.

Minot, L. A. (2003). *Conceiving parenthood: Parenting and the rights of lesbian, gay, bisexual, and transgender people and their children*. San Francisco: International Gay and Lesbian Human Rights Commission.

Morenoff, J. D., Sampson, R. J., & Raudenbush, S. W. (2001). Neighborhood inequality, collective efficacy, and the spatial dynamics of homicide. *Criminology, 39*(3), 517–560.

Nash, J. K. (2002). Neighborhood effects on sense of school coherence and educational behavior in students at risk of school failure. *Children & Schools, 24*(2), 73–89.

National Institute on Media and the Family. (2002, July 8). *Children and advertising*. Retrieved from http://www.mediafamily.org/facts/facts_childadv.shtml

National Research Council. (2005). *Growing up global: The changing transitions to adulthood in developing countries*. Washington, DC: National Academies Press.

National Research Council and National Institute of Medicine. (2000). Neighborhood and community. In J. Shonkoff & D. Phillips (Eds.), *From neurons to neighborhoods: The science of early childhood development* (pp. 328–336). Washington, DC: National Academy Press.

Nayak, A. (2003). 'Through children's eyes': Childhood, place, and the fear of crime. *Geoforum, 34*, 303–315.

Office of the United Nations High Commissioner for Refugees. (2006). *The state of the world's refugees: Human displacement in the new millennium*. Oxford, UK: Oxford University Press.

Plybon, L., Edwards, L., Butler, D., Belgrave, F., & Allison, K. (2003). Examining the link between neighborhood cohesion and school outcomes: The role of support coping among African-American adolescent girls. *Journal of Black Psychology, 29*(4), 393–407.

Popenoe, D. (2008). *Cohabitation, marriage, and child well-being: A cross-national perspective*. Retrieved from http://marriage.rutgers.edu

Pryor, J., Hurtado, S., Saenz, V., Santos, J., & Korn, W. (2007). *The American Freshman: Forty year trends*. Los Angeles: Higher Education Research Institute, UCLA.

Putnam, R. D. (1995). Bowling alone: America's declining social capital. *Journal of Democracy, 6*(1), 65–78.

Raikes, H. A., & Thompson, R. A. (2005). Efficacy and social support as predictors of parenting stress among families in poverty. *Infant Mental Health Journal, 26*(3), 177–190.

Reading, R., Haynes, R., & Shenassa, E. (2005). Neighborhood influences on child injury risk. *Children, Youth, and Environments, 15*(1), 165–185.

Rowlingson, K., & McKay, S. (2006). Lone motherhood and socio-economic disadvantage: Insights from quantitative and qualitative evidence. *Sociological Review, 53*(1), 30–49.

Sampson, R. (2003). The neighborhood context of well-being. *Perspectives in Biology and Medicine, 46*(Suppl.), S53–S64.

Sampson, R., Morenoff, J., & Earls, F. (1999). Beyond social capital: Spatial dynamics of collective efficacy for children. *American Sociological Review, 64*, 633–660.

Sastry, N., & Pebley, A. (2003, April 28). *Neighborhood and family effects on children's health in Los Angeles*. Retrieved from http://www.ccpr.ucla.edu/asp/papers.asp#2003

Schieber, R. A., & Vegega, M. E. (2002). Reducing childhood pedestrian injuries: Summary of a multidisciplinary conference. *Injury Prevention, 8*(Suppl. I), i3–i8.

Scott, T., Taylor, L., & Blakester, A. (2005). *Creating child friendly communities: NAPCAN's approach to preventing child abuse and neglect in Australia*. Retrieved from http://www.engagingcommunities2005.org/abstracts/Scott-Teresa-final.pdf

Shinn, M., & Toohey, S. (2003). Community contexts of human welfare. *Annual Review of Psychology, 54*, 427–459.

Silk, J., Sessa, F., Morris, A., Steinberg, L., & Avenevoli, S. (2004). Neighborhood cohesion as a buffer against hostile maternal parenting. *Journal of Family Psychology, 18*, 135–146.

Slovenia Government Communication Office. (2009, February 15). *Ministry presents policy to increase birthrate*. Retrieved from http://www.ukom.gov.si/eng/slovenia/publications/slovenia-news/3047/3053/

Soubhi, H., Raina, P., & Kohen, D. (2004). Neighborhood, family, and child predictors of childhood injury in Canada. *American Journal of Health Behavior, 28*(5), 397–409.

Tester, J. M., Rutherford, G. W., Wald, Z., & Rutherford, M. W. (2004). A matched case-control study evaluating the effectiveness of speed bumps in reducing child pedestrian injuries. *American Journal of Public Health, 94*, 646–650.

Turcotte, P. (2006, March 14). *Parents with adult children living at home.* Retrieved from http://www.statcan.gc.ca/studies-etudes/11-008/feature-caracteristique/5018786-eng.pdf

United Nations. (2006). *Trends in total migration stock: The 2005 revision.* Department of Social and Economic Affairs, Population Division. New York: United Nations.

United Nations Conference on Trade and Development. (2008). *The least developed countries report 2008.* Geneva: United Nations.

United Nations Population Fund. (2008). *State of the world population 2008: Reaching common ground: Culture, gender, and human rights.* New York: United Nations.

United Nations Statistics Division. (2008, July 21). *Divorces and crude divorce rates by urban/rural residence: 2002–2006.* Retrieved from http://unstats.un.org/unsd/demographic/products/dyb/dyb2006.htm

Velkoff, V. (2002, January 16). *Living arrangements and well-being of the older population: Future research directions.* Retrieved from http://www0.un.org/esa/population/publications/bulletin42_43/velkoff.pdf

Wen, M., & Zhang, X. (2007, February 26). *Neighborhood effects on physical activity: The social and physical environment.* Retrieved from http://www.activelivingresearch.org/alr/node/11460

Widome, R., Sieving, R., Harpin, S., & Hearst, M. (2008). Measuring neighborhood connection and the association with violence in young adolescents. *Journal of Adolescent Health, 43*, 482–489.

Wilcox, P., Quisenberry, N., & Jones, S. (2003). The built environment and community crime risk interpretation. *Journal of Research in Crime and Delinquency, 40*(3), 322–345.

Zani, B., Cicognani, E., & Albanesi, C. (2001). Adolescents' sense of community and feeling of unsafety in the urban environment. *Journal of Community and Applied Social Psychology, 11*, 475–489.

Part II
Setting the Scene

Exploring the Extended Family of Mediterranean Welfare States, or: Did Beveridge and Bismarck Take a Mediterranean Cruise Together?

John Gal

Introduction

The study of welfare states and social policy has enjoyed growing popularity in the last four decades. Emerging from primarily descriptive studies of state-provided welfare, social security, and health institutions and from relatively crude quantitative and qualitative comparative studies, this field has been characterized by a growing level of theorization, richer case study analyses, inclusion of additional sources of welfare provision (nonprofit, market-based, informal, family), and increasingly complex, accurate and up-to-date cross-national comparative analyses (Castles, 2004; Clasen & Siegel, 2007; Ferrera, 2008; Huber & Stephens, 2001; Mabbet & Bolderson, 1999).

One explanation for the growing interest in the welfare state and in various aspects of social policy is the significant role this type of public policy has played in public expenditure in industrialized nations. According to the latest OECD data, net public expenditure on social protection in member countries reached 20.6% of GDP on average in the middle of the first decade of the new millennium (OECD, http://www.oecd.org/dataoecd). In Europe, interest in social policy and, in particular, comparative social policy is motivated by a growing desire on the part of decision-makers in European Union nations to move towards greater coordination and cooperation in the field of social policy (Ferrera, Hemerijick, & Rhodes, 2001; Kleinman, 2002; Kvist & Saari, 2007; Taylor-Gooby, 2002).

A major theme in welfare state research during the last decade and a half has been the growing tendency to create welfare regime typologies, according to which diverse types of welfare regimes are identified (Bambra, 2007; Gough & Wood 2004). The goal of these typologies is to enable scholars to better understand trends and developments within welfare states and to generate credible explanatory variables in order to explain similarities and differences in structures, spending, and

J. Gal (✉)
Paul Baerwald School of Social Work & Social Welfare, Hebrew University of Jerusalem, 91905 Jerusalem, Israel
e-mail: msjgsw@mscc.huji.ac.il

M. Ajzenstadt, J. Gal (eds.), *Children, Gender and Families in Mediterranean Welfare States*, Children's Well-Being: Indicators and Research 2, DOI 10.1007/978-90-481-8842-0_4, © Springer Science+Business Media B.V. 2010

impact (Arts & Gellisen, 2002). In his influential texts, Esping-Andersen (1990, 1999) identified three distinct welfare regimes (the liberal, social-democratic, and corporatist) that differ in the patterns of state, market and household provision of welfare, the degree to which labor is decommodified (i.e., dependence on market forces is weakened), and the impact of welfare state institutions on stratification.

In addition to the three regimes identified by Esping-Andersen, additional welfare regime types have been identified over the years (Arts & Gellisen, 2002). One of these has been variously described as the Latin Rim, the Southern European, or the Mediterranean welfare regime (Ferrera, 1996; Liebfried, 1992; Rhodes, 1997). While the countries identified as belonging to this regime have characteristics that are similar to those of other welfare states, the claim has been that there are nevertheless a number of aspects of welfare state structuring, funding, provision, and results that set them apart. The identification of a unique Mediterranean welfare regime is one starting point for this chapter.

A second point of departure focuses on the two dominant traditions within social policy, those associated with Beveridge and Bismarck (Bonoli, 1997). Given that William Beveridge was only 19-years-old when Otto von Bismarck died in Germany, it is highly unlikely that these two individuals ever actually undertook a Mediterranean tour together. Indeed there is no empirical basis for the claim that the two actually traveled on a cruise ship together, gambling and sunbathing their way through a grand tour of Spanish resorts, Italian ports, Greek islands, and Holy Land sites. Nevertheless, despite the fact that these two gentlemen never made a joint physical appearance in the Mediterranean, the impact of the welfare state legacies associated with their names on the countries in this region is apparent. Even a superficial glance at the welfare regimes in the diverse nations of the Mediterranean appears to indicate that the spirits of Beveridge and Bismarck still haunt the institutions of the welfare states in this region, sometimes appearing solo and at other times in tandem.

My goal in this chapter is to suggest that an extended family of Mediterranean welfare states does indeed exist, that it can offer a useful framework for analysis of welfare states in this geographic region and that we should include in this family a number of nations that have generally been ignored in the discourse on Mediterranean welfare states.[1] More specifically, the claim will be that the conceptual and geographic boundaries of this Mediterranean extended family of welfare states are much less rigid than those generally understood in the notion of a Mediterranean welfare regime and that this family of nations encompasses welfare states modeled on different approaches to the provision of welfare and the structuring of the institutions engaged in provision. The ongoing legacies of Bismarck and Beveridge, as well as other factors, have contributed to differences between

---

[1] I am borrowing the term "family of nations" introduced into the welfare state literature by Castles (1993).

these family members and these differences should not be ignored and sidelined. Nevertheless I will endeavor to underscore a number of features common to members of this extended family of welfare states. Finally, three overarching themes that, in the past and present, appear to indicate the underlying commonalities of Mediterranean welfare states and that can offer potential fruitful avenues for further study will be identified and discussed.

The Extended Family of Mediterranean Welfare States

The notion of a distinctive Mediterranean or Southern European welfare regime emerged shortly after the publication of Esping-Andersen's 1990 book, *The Three Worlds of Welfare Capitalism*. Esping-Andersen included only a single Southern European nation, Italy, in his original schema and it was labeled a corporatist welfare regime.

In a series of studies published in the 1990s in the wake of Esping-Andersen's work, scholars questioned his inclusion of Italy in the corporatist regime type and his exclusion of other southern European welfare states from the analysis (Ferrera, 1996; Liebfried, 1992; Rhodes, 1997). They then went on to suggest that there exists a fourth welfare regime and that this so-called Latin Rim, Southern European, or Mediterranean welfare regime has characteristics which distinguish it from the other welfare regimes. The nations generally included in this regime were Italy, Spain, Portugal, and Greece.

These nations were seen as belonging to a family of nations due not only to their geographic proximity but also due to common historical and cultural legacies. Their common history of relatively recent nondemocratic rule (particularly in the cases of Spain, Portugal, and Greece), the influence of religion (in particular Catholicism) upon diverse aspects of life, not least the family and the provision of welfare, and their seemingly "rudimentary" welfare state systems were underscored as contributing to the need to differentiate these nations from other welfare states (Castles, 1995; Gough, 1996; Liebfried, 1992). More specifically, the three distinctive characteristics of the Mediterranean welfare regime, as identified by Ferrera in the mid-1990s, were the dualism, fragmentation, and ineffectiveness of the social protection system, which often led to marked gaps between segments of society and high levels of poverty within specific geographical or social sectors; the existence of universal (or near universal) health provision by the state alongside a flourishing private health market; and the particularistic-clientelistic form that the welfare state took in these nations (Ferrera, 1996). In addition, a number of observers have underscored the major role of the family, rather than the state, the market or the workplace, as a provider of welfare and care in these countries (Moreno, 2002; Naldini, 2003). Looking at issues of social expenditure and the type of financing predominant in various welfare states, Bonoli (1997) added two additional features of the Mediterranean family of nations that depict some of these characteristics from another perspective – low levels of social expenditure combined with an adherence to the Bismarckian tendency to prefer contribution-funded and income-related benefits over the use of tax-funded flat-rated transfer programs.

Despite Esping-Andersen's (1999) later rejection of this attempt to identify a distinctive Mediterranean regime, a number of studies undertaken in the years since have found varying degrees of support for the model. This is the case with regard to policies adopted by the nations affiliated to this regime and their consequences (Aassve, Mazzuco, & Mencarini, 2005; Arnstein, Mazzuco, & Mencarini, 2005; Chesnais, 1996; Ferreira, 2008; Fouarge & Layte, 2005; Mâitre, Nolan, & Whelan, 2005; Muffels & Fouarge, 2004; Ogg, 2005; Trifiletti, 1999; Tsakloglou & Papadopolous, 2002), to certain characteristics of these societies (Guiliano, 2007), to the self-perceptions of the citizens of these countries (Eikemo, Bambra, Judge, & Ringdal, 2008), and to their attitudes to diverse welfare state issues within them (Ginn & Fast, 2006).

In more contemporary welfare state research discourse, regime terminology and particularly the regime typology formulated by Esping-Andersen has been subjected to conceptual and methodological criticism (Arts & Gellisen, 2002). In addition to the claims that the original Esping-Andersen typology ignored additional regime types and that it failed to take into account fundamental issues of gender (Lewis, 1997; Orloff, 1993), critics have found fault with various methodological aspects of his original analysis (Bambra, 2006; Scruggs & Allan, 2006) and with the over-emphasis upon cash transfers rather than social services of different kinds (Bambra, 2005; Jensen, 2008). More damning, perhaps, has been the assertion that the assumption that there is any dominant approach to welfare provision in a single regime or that there is any coherence in social policy in a single country is extremely problematic (Kasza, 2002). Linked to this is the sense that changes over time lead to qualitative and quantitative changes in the structuring of welfare states and a diluting of the significant differences that existed between the regimes in the past. Factors such as globalization, movement towards a European Social Model by European welfare states, and peer pressure upon welfare state laggards within the EU to increase social spending and achieve standards of coverage and benefit generosity on a par with a European norm, appear to be major contributing factors to this process.

The Southern European welfare regime, it seems, is particularly susceptible to these political and social transformations. Progress towards European integration, marked economic and labor market changes, and welfare institution restructuring in the nations of Southern Europe have tended to blur some of the more distinctive differences between these and other countries in Europe (Morlino, 2002). The Europeanization of Spain, Portugal, Italy, and Greece appear to have pushed them much closer to an emerging European Social Model (Andreotti et al., 2001; Cousins, 2005; Guillén, Álvarez, & Adão e Silva, 2003; Kvist & Saari, 2007). Despite these developments, there still appears to remain a number of distinctive characteristics that differentiate welfare states in the Mediterranean region from those to their north in Europe and across the seas in America and Australasia (Moreno, 2006; Vogel, 2004).

Enlarging the Mediterranean Family

Traditionally, the focus of research and debate concerning the Mediterranean family of nations has been on a small number of countries in Southern Europe (Spain, Portugal, Italy, and Greece), all of which were members of the EU 15. Nevertheless, some observers have tended to extend the nations included in this family of nations to encompass others. This is particularly the case due to moves in recent years to expand membership of the European Union. Alongside the major eastward direction of extension of the union, a southward process also occurred. Two Mediterranean island nations, Cyprus and Malta, were the principle beneficiaries of this extension and in recent literature tend to be incorporated in the Southern European grouping of welfare states (Grasselli, Montesi, & Iannone, 2006). Turkey, a candidate country and potential member of the EU, has of course been the subject of much debate within European Union nations (Manning, 2007). As such, its welfare and social protection systems have been the subject of growing interest and some observers both within Turkey and abroad have also included this country in discussion of the Mediterranean family of nations (Buğra & Keyder, 2006; Gough, 1996; Saraceno, 2002).

Israel has not usually been included in the literature on the Mediterranean family of nations. Not being a candidate country for membership in the European Union (though affiliated to the EU in various ways), it has not generated much interest in welfare state-related discussions within Europe. Moreover, there is much uncertainty and contention regarding the relevance of existing welfare state typologies to the Israeli case. While some observers have portrayed Israel as exhibiting characteristics similar to those of a corporatist welfare regime (Okun, Oliver, & Khait-Marelly, 2007), others have emphasized its social-democratic tendencies in the past and its current move towards a liberal welfare regime type (Doron, 2001; Gal, 2004). Its affinity to other Mediterranean nations has seldom emerged in the literature (but, see Doron, 2003).

To what degree do the countries discussed above (Cyprus, Malta, Turkey, and Israel) have anything in common with the more traditional members of the Mediterranean family of nations (Spain, Portugal, Italy, and Greece)? Geographic proximity to the Mediterranean Sea is, of course, the most obvious common denominator with regard to all of these nations (with the exception of Portugal). However, neither geographic proximity, nor a common history of wars and domination by ancient empires, or, for that matter, a love of olive oil and good bread make a family of nations as far as welfare and social protection are concerned.

Indeed, a cursory glance at these nations appears to offer little support for the claim that they belong to a single (albeit extended) family of welfare states. They are distinguishable in a number of key demographic, social, economic, political, and cultural features that would appear to undermine any effort to find a degree of commonality between them.

Clearly the religious affiliation and cultural heritage of these nations are diverse. Some of these countries, particularly those that comprise the Latin Rim of Western Europe, are predominantly Roman Catholic. The vast majority of Turks are Muslims

while Greek Orthodoxy is the religious affiliation of most of the inhabitants of
Greece and Cyprus. Finally, Israel is officially a Jewish state though its population
comprises a significant minority of Arabs, most of whom are Muslims.

Demographically, these nations include countries which diverge quite dramatically with regard to size and composition. The total population in these countries
ranges from a low of less than a million in the island states of Cyprus and Malta, to
a high of 73 million in Turkey, with its land mass of 780,580 km^2. While in some of
these countries, the urban population comprises a very high proportion of the population (in Malta and in Israel it is over 90%), in other nations, such as Greece and
Turkey, over a third of the population still reside in rural areas. The Mediterranean
welfare states have fertility rates and proportions of children and the elderly in the
population that are among both the highest and the lowest among welfare states.
Spain and Italy are exemplars of welfare states afflicted with particularly low fertility rates and that consequently have a low proportion of children and high proportion
of elders. Thus, in Spain and Italy the total fertility rates are currently 1.38 and 1.32
respectively, well below replacement level fertility, while the proportion of children
under the ages of 14 in these countries is 14.5 and 14.1%, much less than the mean
in the European Union. Finally, the proportion of individuals over the age of 65 is
nearing a fifth of the population in these countries. By contrast, in the two demographic outliers among the Mediterranean welfare states – Turkey and Israel, both
the fertility rates and the proportion of children in the total population are higher
than in most other welfare states, while the proportion of the elderly is lower. In
Turkey, while dropping in recent decades the fertility rate is still high at 2.19, children comprise 28.3% of the population and the proportion of elderly is only 5.9%. In
Israel, the fertility rate is even higher than that of Turkey – 2.88, children comprise
28% of the population, and the elderly are currently 10% of the overall population.

Similarly, the standards of living and social conditions of the inhabitants of the
various Mediterranean nations differ significantly. This is particularly the case when
comparing Turkey to some of the welfare states to its west. Thus, while GDP per
capita in Spain and Italy are in excess of 20,000 EUR, the per capita level in Turkey
is only 4,400 EUR. The GDP per capita of Malta, the nation with the second lowest GDP per capita of these countries, is 14,200 EUR. These differences in living
standards are reflected in other social indices. For example, net secondary school
enrollment is over 90% in most of the Mediterranean nations but drops to 85% in
Malta and to 66% in Turkey. Similarly, while the proportion of homes owning a
personal computer is over 40% in most of these countries and indeed is over 60%
in Israel, in Turkey it is only 12%. Finally, while the labor market participation rate
is high in some of these nations, reaching 69.6% in Cyprus, it is as low as 54.8% in
Malta and 45.9% in Turkey (European Commission, 2006; Eurostat, 2007).

Looking beyond these more general issues, the structure of the welfare state of
the nations discussed here differ and, in particular, reflect distinctive legacies. The
two social policy legacies that dominate the literature are those associated with Otto
von Bismarck and with William Beveridge. Bismarckian social policies originated
in the policies adopted by the German Chancellor in the 1880s to establish a state-
run social insurance program that would enable him to undercut the demands of

the labor movement and ensure political stability in the country by offering workers insurance to protect against the threats of old age and invalidity (Alber, 1986; Zöllner, 1982). Evoking the insurance principle, these policies required contributions on the part of workers and their employers in addition to state subsidies with the administration typically entrusted to semi-autonomous and often jointly (employer and employee) run social funds. As such, these policies have primarily sought to provide job and income security for male workers. Thus, they have traditionally privileged employees, seeking to ensure that the social protection programs reflect the living standards of the participants, while offering much weaker protection to individuals, particularly women, outside the labor market. In practice, Bismarckian social policies have tended to provide earnings-related benefits for employees that are funded primarily by employers and employees with entitlement generally linked to a contributory history. While welfare states influenced by this legacy will have additional noncontributory programs for individuals in need, with no links to the labor market, the emphasis will be upon income maintenance, a preference for contributions as a primary source of funding, and marked differences between benefits to diverse social groups and between individuals who have labor market experience and those who do not (Palier & Martin, 2007; Bonoli, 1997).

In contrast, Beveridgean social policy is influenced by the proposals included in the document prepared by a committee headed by William Beveridge and submitted to the British government in 1942 during the Second World War (Hills, Ditch, & Glennerster 1994). While not discarding social insurance notions, the Beveridgean approach to social protection identifies alleviation of poverty as the main goal of social policy and seeks to structure an inclusive social protection system that focuses on a wide range of needs and contingencies ("cradle to grave") and that is based on coverage of the entire population. Here need and residence are the dominant criterion for qualification rather than contribution. Programs based on this approach to social policy offer either universal or means-tested benefits that do not distinguish between prior income levels of eligible recipients with regard to benefit level but offer a similar benefit to all. As such, funding tends to come primarily from general taxation and benefits are generally flat-rate and not earnings-related (Bonoli, 1997).

While pure Bismarckian or Beveridgean welfare states have never existed, and certainly do not exist today, social policy scholarship does distinguish between the structuring of social protection systems that have been influenced predominantly by one of these legacies. Two tools can offer a relatively straight forward means to applying this understanding to comparative analysis. Welfare states influenced by the Bismarckian legacy will presumably be those in which a greater proportion of funding for social protection programs is based upon contributions from employers and employees and in which alleviation of poverty among nonworking individuals of working age is left to the nongovernment sector or is a relatively new development, primarily a consequence of the external influence of European integration. By contrast, a Beveridgean legacy should result in a greater tendency to fund social protection programs through general tax revenues and an early adoption of residual safety net programs for the poor. Table 1 presents data on the Mediterranean welfare states with regard to sources of funding and the existence of safety net programs.

Table 1 Countries by
proportion of contributions
and safety nets

Country	Contributions as a proportion of social protection funding	Existence of a longstanding national safety net program
Cyprus	37.3	+
Israel	45.5	+
Malta	64.2	+
Portugal	47.5	+/−[a]
Italy	56	−[b]
Greece	60.8	−
Spain	67.2	−[c]
Turkey	n.a.	−

[a]National program introduced in 2003.
[b]No national program, local initiatives.
[c]Nonuniform local programs.

Of the eight countries, two, Israel and Cyprus, appear to have been clearly influenced by the Beveridgean legacy (Doron, 1994; Shekeris, 1998). In both, contributions comprise a relatively low proportion of social protection funding and they both have long standing safety net programs. Not surprisingly, the social welfare systems were modeled closely on the British system during periods of British colonial rule and in its wake. In contrast, Greece, Italy, and Spain are three nations clearly influenced by the Bismarckian legacy (Venieris, 1997). Contributions comprise a major proportion of funding for social protection and safety net programs either do not exist or are partial and lack a national statutory basis (Matsaganis, Ferrera, Capucha, & Moreno, 2003). While it has some social assistance programs, Turkey lacks any comprehensive safety net infrastructure (Buğra & Keyder, 2006). Malta and Portugal appear to be more hybrid cases. While contributions comprise a major proportion of social protection funding in Malta, this is a relatively new phenomenon, and the country has a long-standing safety net program modeled on the British system (Grasselli et al., 2006). In the Portuguese case, historical analysis has indicated the impact of both British and German influences on social security structuring (Guibentif, 1997). In this country, there has been a marked increase in state funding for social protection in recent years and a national safety net program was introduced in 1997 on a national scale (Guillén et al., 2003).

Despite these and other differences between the various Mediterranean welfare states and the specific features of each of the nations, a review of diverse quantitative data indicates that there is some basis for the claim that these nations do share a number of common features that distinguish them from other welfare states, in addition to the characteristics that draw so many North American and North European tourists to their shores.

The charts below compare the Mediterranean (in gray columns) nations to countries representative of other welfare regimes (in black columns). Seen in a comparative perspective, the Mediterranean welfare states are generally characterized by relatively low levels of economic production, with GDP per capita figures

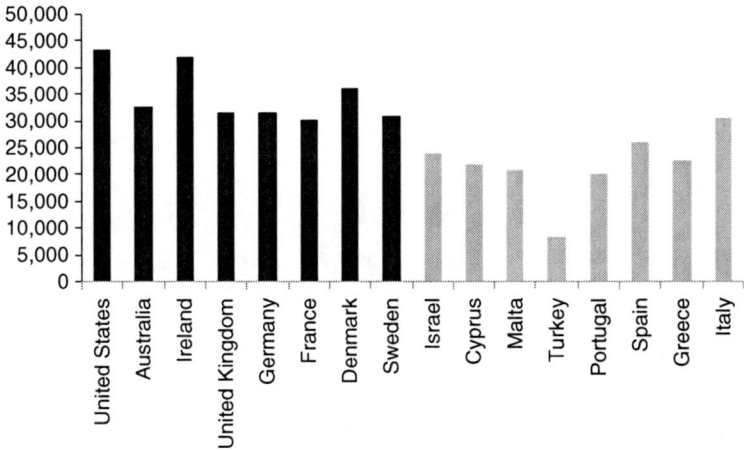

Chart 1 GDP per capita in Mediterranean and other welfare states, 2006 (current prices, PPP, $US) (Source: IMF World Economic Outlook Database)

lower than in most advanced industrial societies (see Chart 1). This is particularly marked in the cases of Turkey, Portugal, and Malta. An examination of the effort spent on social protection programs in these countries, as measured by the levels of social expenditure as a proportion of GDP (see Chart 2), indicates that, while most of the Mediterranean nations have undergone a catch-up process of growing social spending in recent decades, expenditure levels generally remain lower than those in the social-democratic and corporatist welfare states and higher than those in liberal welfare states such as the United States.

Low levels of labor market participation, particularly that of women, has long been identified as a feature of Mediterranean welfare states and has been linked to

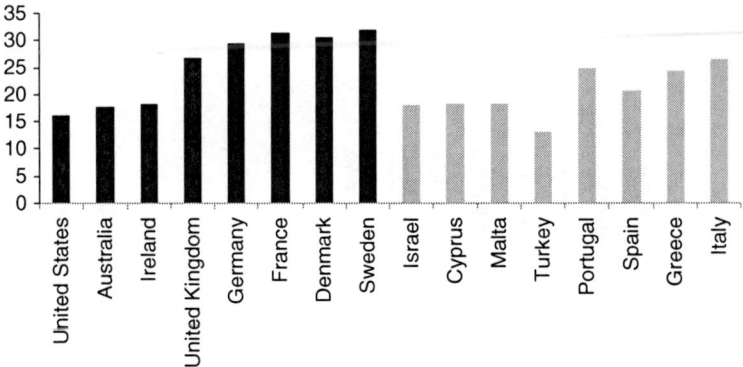

Chart 2 Total social expenditure as % of GDP (Sources: Australia, USA – OECD, 2003; Israel – National Insurance Institute of Israel, 2003; Turkey – www.un.org; All other states – Eurostat, 2005 (Portugal – 2004))

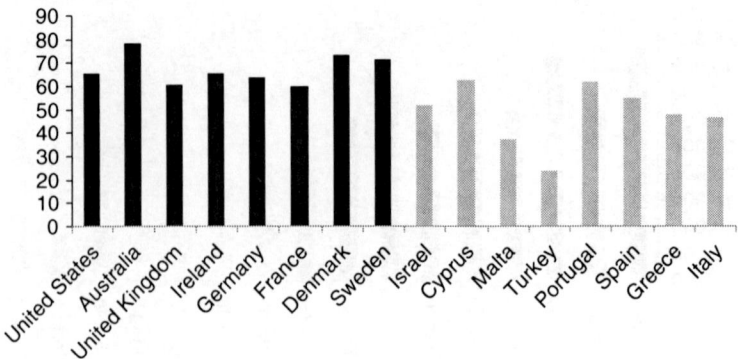

Chart 3 Female labor market participation* (*age group – 15–64; Sources: Australia – OECD, 2006; Israel – Central Bureau of Statistic, 2007; All other states – Eurostat, 2007 (Turkey, USA – 2006))

the nature of economic development and the dominance of the male-breadwinner model associated with these countries (Chart 3). Findings indicate that this is still true to a certain degree in most of these nations and that, with the exception of Portugal and Cyprus, these nations still have relatively low levels of female labor market participation, that is on a par with or even lower than those in corporatist welfare states.

An inevitable consequence of relatively low levels of social spending and low labor market participation rates in the Mediterranean welfare states is the limited ability of the welfare state to deal effectively with poverty levels and inequality. Chart 4 below offers evidence of this. Comparative data on at-risk poverty levels (set at 60% of the median income) indicate that the proportion of the population at risk of poverty in Mediterranean nations is higher than that in most other European welfare

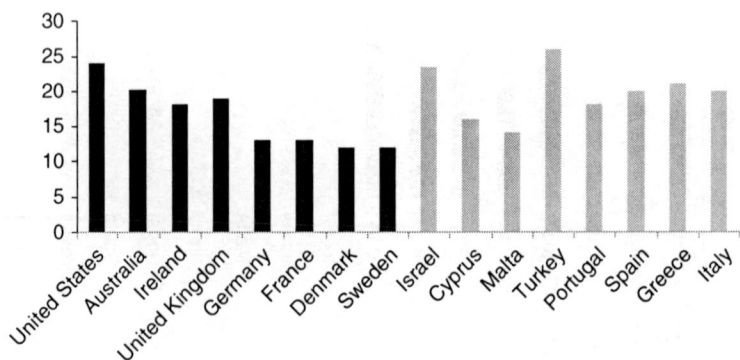

Chart 4 At-risk-poverty (60%) (Sources: Australia – Luxemburg Income Study, 2003; USA – Luxemburg Income Study, 2004; Israel – Luxemburg Income Study, 2001; All other states – Eurostat, 2006 (Turkey – 2003))

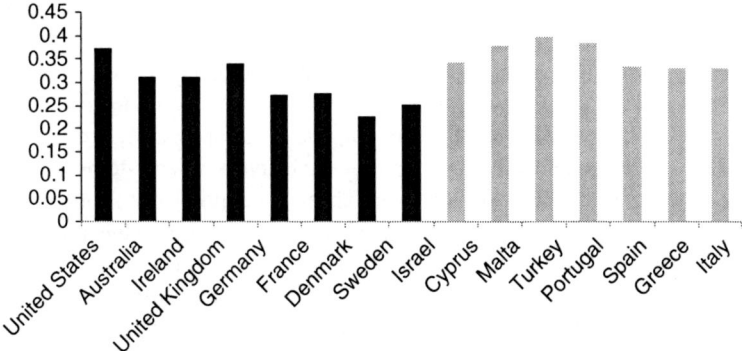

Chart 5 Gini coefficients (Sources: Turkey – The World Bank, 2004; All other countries – Luxemburg Income Study, 2000 (AU 2003, DK 2004, IL 2001, UK 1999, USA 2004); Malta – no data available)

states and equal or higher than that in liberal welfare states. Similarly, inequality levels measured by the Ginni coefficient (see Chart 5) show that social gaps remain high in the extended family of Mediterranean welfare states, once again apparently indicating an inability on the part of the welfare state to successfully overcome social gaps through redistribution.

The Contours of an Extended Family of Mediterranean Welfare States

Clearly differences, sometimes very marked, distinguish between the various welfare states within the Mediterranean region and indeed, at least in the cases of Italy and Spain, between geographical regions within these nations themselves (Fargion, 1997). Nevertheless, the figures above do offer grounds for a more compelling argument that a distinctive extended family of Mediterranean welfare states does exist and can serve as the basis for an enhanced understanding of the dynamics of welfare and social developments within these countries.

Viewed from a historical perspective, the commonalities of these countries (and their divergence from other welfare regime models) would appear to be linked to the fact that, in contrast to other welfare states, all underwent relatively delayed processes of industrialization and modernization. With the exception of some pockets in Italy and Spain, agriculture remained a major source of employment and domestic product in these countries long after this was no longer the case in other welfare states. Full-scale industrialization occurred significantly later in these nations than in most of Western Europe or North America, reaching levels comparable to other advanced capitalist nations in Europe only in the 1960s and 1970s. This process generally involved the decline in relative importance of agriculture, and the shift of employment and production from this sector to industry and services and marked changes in the organization of capital (Hudson & Lewis, 1984). It also consisted of a move from primarily autarkic economies in many of these countries, particularly those with authoritarian regimes, to a more globalized economy with high levels of foreign investment, know-how and tourism (Sapelli, 1995; Williams, 1984).

While all of these countries have distinctive political histories, all differ from most other welfare states in the fact that they have democratic systems that are characterized by either discontinuity or have existed for a relatively short time period. These are nations that have recent histories of authoritarian rule (Greece, Italy, Portugal, Spain, and Turkey) or (in the cases of Malta, Cyprus, and Israel) of colonial dominance until well into the middle of the twentieth century. In most of these welfare states, ongoing internal ethnic, political or regional strife, or external military struggles have threatened to undermine the democratic structure of the unitary state. As a result, democracy within these countries has been much more fragile than that in other welfare states. Consequently, the political systems in all these countries appear to be less stable, more prone to crisis, and often grossly ineffective. Not surprisingly perhaps, Kurth (1993, p. 27) has described the political systems of Southern Europe as the "least legitimate" in the European Community. This would appear to be the case in all of the nations within the Mediterranean extended family.

Some observers have underscored the fact that the state in these countries is, both stronger and weaker than in other welfare states. While low levels of welfare provision and institutions highly vulnerable to partisan pressure (Ferrera, 1996) are evidence of its weakness, the state in these nations has sought to play a major role in regulating most spheres of social life and in controlling major social and economic institutions (Andreotti et al., 2001). One indication of this is the structuring and functioning of bureaucracies in these countries. Sotiropoulos (2004a) has noted that bureaucracies in the four South European states are characterized by enduring party politicization of the higher echelons of the civil service, patronage patterns of recruitment and an uneven distribution of human resources in the state sector, an emphasis on formalism and legalism and a lack of traditional administrative elite. Again, it would appear that most or even all of these traits are to be found in the other Mediterranean welfare states as well.

Late industrialization and modernity, a recent memory of colonial rule or non-democratic regimes, ongoing threats to the political and social system, and weak central states and ineffective public bureaucracies have implications for the funding, structuring and functioning of welfare states. These characteristics have limited the resources available for funding a comprehensive social protection system and have created difficulties in the administration of established programs. Late industrialization inevitably influenced the formation of the working class and the strength of broad-based working class political and labor market movements, which traditionally formed the backbone of pro-universal welfare state coalitions in many countries. A lack of democratic legitimacy or stability has encouraged the manipulation of social welfare programs in order to gain political support while simultaneously undermining efforts to engage in long-term social welfare planning. Ethnic and regional tension, along with external threats to the sovereignty of these nations, has not only served to divert resources to other fields of state activity, such as military readiness or internal security, but also to undermine support for the introduction of universal social protection programs that cut across ethnic, regional, and class lines. Finally, the legacies of authoritarianism and colonialism had inevitable repercussions on public attitudes to social protection policies adopted by elites. In particular, these legacies have either created backlashes against the values of these regimes or, by contrast, have created path dependencies that have lingering impacts on welfare state structuring.

However, beyond these common political and economic developments, three additional themes appear to underlie welfare state formulation in the Mediterranean countries and distinguish them from other welfare states. These themes are religion, the family, and the persistence of clientelistic-particularistic forms of welfare.

Religion

Religion has, of course, been regarded as a factor in determining economic behavior even since the publication of Max Weber's *The Protestant Ethic and the Spirit of Capitalism* in the first decade of the twentieth century (Weber, 1958). Yet, apart from a few notable exceptions (Castles, 1994; Heidenheimer, 1983; Wilensky, 1981), the role of religion in the development, structuring, and functioning of welfare states has only recently attracted significant theoretical attention (Algun & Cahuc, 2006; Cnaan & Boddie, 2002; Kahl, 2005; Manow, 2004; Manow & van Kersbergen, 2006; Opielka, 2008; van Oorschot, 2007). This contemporary literature perceives religion and religious belief as a variable that can contribute to understanding divergence and commonality between welfare states. It distinguishes between various religious denominations and seeks to unravel the links between religion, social cleavages, political structures, and welfare state institutions. This literature also identifies diverse avenues through which religion has, and continues, to influence welfare state institutions. These appear to have existed both separately and in congruence in the past within nations that have become welfare states, and they often continue to serve as conduits through which religion has an impact on the functioning of social protection services in the present. These avenues consist of organizational and cultural legacies, contemporary public attitudes, the role of political parties affiliated with religious organizations, the influence of religious hierarchies on political elites, and the impact of the provision of core social welfare services by religious organizations upon state willingness to offer similar services.

While religion has been discussed in some of the literature concerning Southern European welfare states (Ferrera, 1996; Liebfried, 1992), this has generally taken the form of claims that the Catholic affiliation of the majority of the populations in these countries can perhaps contribute to explaining some of the features of these nations, in particular those pertaining to issues of gender and the lack of uniform and comprehensive social safety net programs (Gough, 1996). Nevertheless, the employment of religion as an explanatory variable in the literature on Southern European welfare states has been limited for a number of reasons. Among others, these explanations have had restricted impact on the debate because of the fact that only three of the four Southern European nations are indeed Catholic (most Greeks are affiliated with the Orthodox Church). Also problematic is the fact that Catholicism appears to be related to welfare state structuring in nations beyond Southern Europe as well and therefore is not a unique feature of the Mediterranean countries (see, for example, Castles, 1994). For example, the existence of major Christian Democratic political parties established on the basis of Catholic thinking and a significant proportion of Catholics in the populations of Germany and the Netherlands are features that have been identified as being influential in the specific development of welfare states in these nations (van Kersbergen, 1995). Finally, the fact that a dramatic process of secularization appears to have been underway in at least one of the Mediterranean nations (Spain) during the last few decades (Requena, 2005) would appear to undermine any effort to link religion to social policy development in this country.

Nevertheless, a re-examination of the way in which religion, albeit viewed in a broader sense, has been a force in the forging of welfare states in the Mediterranean region is warranted. It is suggested here that the role of religion can take two seemingly contradictory forms in the structuring of welfare states and social policy. It can, as an organizational entity or a set of cultural values, play a major role in initiating the establishment of social welfare institutions or in the actual formulation of social policies and the identification of their goals. Or, as in Spain during the post-Franco era and in Israel during the pre-state Palestine period, social policy can be formulated as a reaction against religion by political actors supported by anti-religious social groups. In both cases, religion or religious cleavages are factors that cannot be ignored in the analysis of welfare states and is particularly the case for Mediterranean nations.

In all the eight nations in this extended family of welfare states, religion has been a major source of values and organized religion has enjoyed institutional and political power during the period of welfare state formulation and beyond. Even in those nations where the role of the Church has waned, the ongoing legacy of Church-influenced social welfare structures continues, while the formulation of more contemporary policies is, as noted above, often seen as a reaction to the values or power of organized religion in the past. In most of these nations, religious affiliation remains particularly strong and is certainly stronger than that in most other European welfare states. Indeed, in many of the Mediterranean nations the separation of state and religion is nonexistent or, at the very least, contested (see, for example, Danopolous, 2004 and Makrides & Molokotos-Liederman, 2004 on the Greek case and Falzon, 2007 on the Maltese case). As such, religion continues to influence social policy through formal political representation (Turkey and Israel), the activities of religious social welfare organizations, via public attitudes, or due to the more discreet impact of elite interaction.

While the populations of the Mediterranean nations adhere to diverse religious denominations, none of these countries has ever had a major Protestantism foothold. This is crucial due to the growing recognition of the influence of Protestantism, be it Lutheran or Reformed Protestantism, upon the structuring of welfare states.

Manow (2004) has, for example, underscored the differential impact of Lutheranism upon the Scandinavian welfare states and that of Reformed Protestantism upon Anglo-Saxon nations, such as the United States. Though the diversity of religious affiliations in the Mediterranean countries and the specific contours of the political and social institutions in these countries inevitably lead to distinctive configurations of the role of religion in the welfare state, the fact that these are all non-Protestant nations clearly limits the appeal of values and policies that have been directly attributed to the influence of Protestant tenets.

Moreover, not only are the nations comprising the extended family of Mediterranean welfare states non-Protestant but it would appear that a case can be made for the claim that there are certain similarities in the manner in which poverty, poverty alleviation, and the role of the State in dealing with issues of social welfare are perceived by adherents to Catholicism, the Orthodox Church, Islam, and Judaism and that these differ from those of Protestants. Prominent among these is the role that community faith-based social welfare organizations have in dealing with social needs and, in particular, poverty (Bugra, 2007; Jaffe, 1992; Symeonidou, 1997). These organizations, which have been seen as a reflection of an adherence to concepts such as *caritas*, *zakat*, and *zedakah* in the various nations (Dean & Khan, 1997; Kahl, 2005; Kuran, 2003; Sherwin, 2000), can be seen as influencing the manner in which Mediterranean welfare states perceive the need for, or the generosity of, state-run safety net programs. While in some of the nations this has led to the lack of such programs, in others there is a marked emphasis on local provision of this support or of very limited support by existing national state-administered programs, as these are seen to complement existing provision by community faith-based nonprofits. In sum, it would appear that in the nations of the extended family of Mediterranean welfare states religion has, and generally continues, to exert a marked influence on the structuring and functioning of welfare state institutions, to a degree uncommon in other welfare states or in a manner that is unique to this family of nations.

Family

A second issue that has particular resonance in all the welfare states in the Mediterranean is that of the family. While the Mediterranean nations have long been seen as "familialistic" countries, more recent research has sought to investigate the more specific contours of the ways in which the welfare state, the family, and the market interact within these nations and the implications of this for households, gender relations, and for the structuring of the welfare state (see, for example, Ajzenstadt & Gal, 2001; Naldini & Saraceno, 2008; Kiliç, 2008; Moreno, 2004; Prince Cook, 2009). Indeed, despite ongoing changes in female labor market participation and the introduction of some social protection programs and social services that facilitate a better family/work balance, it would appear that the family unit in Mediterranean nations continues to play a distinctive role, and to take a form, that differs from the norm in other welfare states. In a recent work on the subject, Manuela Naldini (2003) coined the term "a family/kinship solidarity model" to describe these nations. In doing so, she sought to underscore the enduring sense of strong and extended family obligations in these societies along with the notion that care work remains a family responsibility. In addition, she noted the relatively low level of state support for families with children in the Mediterranean welfare states.

The centrality of the family in Mediterranean welfare states is, of course, not unrelated to the major role that religion has played in these nations, and continues to play in many of them. Indeed, as in the case of social assistance, there does appear to be a dividing line between the more "individualistic" Protestant ethic and a more "communalistic" ethic, that emphasizes the importance of marriage and leads to more intense family ties and responsibilities, which is more predominant among the Catholic, Orthodox, Islamic, and Jewish societies of the Mediterranean (Greeley, 1989; Martin, 1997).

Be it religion, the late modernization that characterizes Mediterranean nations, or other cultural or societal variables, it is clear that there are marked differences between these nations and most other welfare states (with the possible exception of Ireland) in the way in which the family is perceived and the form that it takes (Moreno, 2006). Marriage is more institutionalized in these nations and family solidarity more important than in other welfare states, particularly as compared to those in central and northern Europe (Guerrero & Naldini, 1997). This is reflected in comparative statistical data which indicates that the proportion of marriages in these countries remains particularly high while alternative cohabitation arrangements are still uncommon. Similarly, the number of single parent households is generally much lower in the extended family of Mediterranean welfare states than in Social-Democratic or Liberal welfare states. Finally, the age until which children remain in their parents' household appears to be higher in the Mediterranean nations (Toren, 2003; Vogel, 2003).

As noted above, fertility rates within the Mediterranean extended family are both the lowest and the highest among welfare states. Fertility rates are particularly low in Spain, Italy, and Greece and high in Turkey and Israel. There are diverse factors that have been identified as having had an impact upon the fertility rates in these nations. While high levels of fertility can be linked to lower educational capital in some of these nations, the lack of extensive pro-family social policies, labor market integration of women and the consequent opportunity costs involved in childbirth have been regarded as a determinant in the low fertility levels of Spanish and Italian women (Guerrero & Naldini, 1997). In those Mediterranean nations with a recent legacy of authoritarian regimes that actively promoted pro-natal policies, a lack of pro-family policies and low fertility rates are interpreted as a reaction to the policies of that period (Naldini, 2003). Strange as it may seem, the dominant role of religion in the past or present in the Mediterranean nations, is apparently one of the factors that has apparently contributed to both the low and high fertility rates. In some cases, particularly in Catholic nations, the lack of divorce laws until much later than other welfare states appears to have discouraged early marriage and thus contributed to the existence of smaller families (Guerrero & Naldini, 1997). By contrast, adherence to the Muslim and Jewish faiths appears to encourage higher fertility rates, a phenomenon particularly common among more traditional and lesser educated inhabitants of Turkey and Israel (İşik & Pinarcioglu, 2006). Similarly, the impact of religion upon social policy and specifically the introduction of generous child benefits for large families has been claimed to be one of the factors contributing to high levels of fertility in Israel (Manski & Meyshar, 2002).

The centrality of the family in the Mediterranean nations and a strong sense of solidarity within the extended family that is dominant within these societies has, of course, significant implications for the ways in which social needs are dealt with and hence upon the structuring and functioning of welfare states. In particular, the existence of strong family support networks and an acceptance of care responsibilities by family members (primarily women) lessen the pressure upon states to deal with diverse needs. The centrality of the family enables welfare states to rely on the family as an alternative to either state or market provision of care. This dependence thereby limits, or deflects, state spending on services and benefits intended to deal with these specific needs. Thus, we find that despite a marked growth in female labor market participation in most of these countries, care for the young, the sick, and the elderly is still very much the responsibility of the family (Andreotti et al., 2001; Grasselli et al., 2006; Moreno, 2006). As such, unpaid care remains the domain of married women or daughters, particularly in the case of the infirmed elderly. Family funded care is provided mainly by immigrant caregivers (Akalin, 2007; Da Roit, 2007). This ongoing manifestation of intergenerational family care is linked to existing social norms and to a lack of adequate family friendly social services and benefits that could offer state-provided alternatives to these tasks or encourage a more equitable gendered division of labor within the family. Not surprisingly perhaps, one observer has employed the term – "superwomen" to describe the role of women in these welfare states due to the need to combine work and family responsibilities (Moreno, 2002). Clearly, an understanding of the workings of the welfare states included within the Mediterranean extended family of nations cannot be achieved without a better understanding of the nexus between state, family, and market with regard to welfare provision (Martin, 1997).

Clientelism-Particularism

A characteristic long associated with the Mediterranean nations has been that of clientelism. In particular, it has been claimed that politics in these nations is dominated (or, at the very least, tainted) by patron–client relations that entail the provision of tangible resources in return for political support (Eisenstadt & Roniger, 1984). In the past, discussion of clientelism in Mediterranean countries was typically couched in culturalistic terms and linked to their delayed process of modernization and democratization in comparison to other capitalist societies (Weingrod, 1968). These studies, however, tended to view clientelistic relations narrowly, they failed to account for change over time in the form that these relations have taken, or to satisfactorily explain the re-emergence, or the persistence, of clientelism in post-industrial and fully democratized society.

Renewed interest in the subject of clientelism in political science and sociological literature in recent years (Roniger, 2004) has resulted in more nuanced definitions of the phenomenon, more diverse applications of the term, and efforts to better contextualize clientelism and to view it in a historical perspective. These developments can offer interesting avenues for seeking commonalities between Mediterranean nations and a better understanding of the workings of these welfare states.

Current approaches to clientelism and patronage view these as potential strategies that can be employed in diverse forms and in various political settings and structures. Piattoni's definition exemplifies this approach. Clientelism and patronage, she notes "are strategies for the acquisition, maintenance and aggrandizement of political power, on the part of patrons, and strategies for the protection and promotion of their interests, on the part of clients, and their deployment is driven by given sets of incentives and disincentives" (2001, p. 2). Seen in this manner, clientelism can take a wide variety of forms. It may take the form of personal relations between a politician and an individual seeking a specific favor, but it may also emerge as reciprocal relations between politicians, political parties or political elites and social groups or social categories that can vary in size and characteristics. Mass clientelism will typically take the form of more formalized relations and be realized through the passage of laws that serve the particular needs of the members of the group. This approach to clientelism seeks to emphasize that clientelistic relations reflect the decision on the part of both patrons and clients to choose this strategy as a means to further their interests and that, if these goals are not furthered, it will be abandoned or restructured. Not only does this approach to clientelism underscore that the employment of this strategy is a consequence of decisions of both individuals and groups (patrons and clients), it also notes that clientelistic strategies, as a means of furthering interests in the political sphere, are path dependent. Drawing upon work by Shefter (1994) on the ways in which political parties structure their appeal to voters, clientelism is seen as a political approach which, while changing in form and effect, can be linked to the timing and form of state-building and, in particular, of mass political mobilization.

Given the centrality of welfare state services and benefits to the needs of individuals and families, the importance of welfare state institutions as a source of employment, and the sheer size of expenditure devoted to these institutions, it is hardly surprising that these have often been the focus of clientelistic relations. Ferrera (1996) has identified this as a feature of Southern European welfare states, emphasizing the scope and intensity of particularistic, rather than universal and impartial, rules and practices in the welfare bureaucracies of these nations. Indeed it would appear that clientelism is a characteristic of all the nations in the extended family of Mediterranean welfare states and remains a critical tool in any effort to understand the nature of these welfare states (Davaki & Mossialos, 2005; Eisenstadt & Roniger, 1984; Hopkin & Mastropaolo, 2001; Mitchell, 2002; Rocha & Araújo, 2007).

While it exists in all the Mediterranean welfare states, clientelism takes on different forms in the various nations and its intensity and relevance varies between them, between regions within them, and over time. In some cases, such as that of Spain, Portugal and Greece, clientelism focuses on the provision of jobs within the higher or lower echelons of the bureaucracies engaged in welfare provision (Ferrera, 1996; Featherstone, 2005; Hopkin, 2001; Sotiropoulos, 2004b). In others, particularly Malta and Turkey, it can take the form of more direct distribution of resources by local political leaders (Heper, 2002; Mitchell, 2002; Mullard & Pirotta, 2008). Sophisticated practices intended to influence the decisions of administrative bodies, such as those determining eligibility to disability benefits, are another type of clientelism, often linked to the Italian welfare state. Finally, as is the case in the Israeli welfare state, legislation that favors the particularlistic interests of the members of specific social categories can be adopted at the behest of political parties (Charbit, 2003).

Whatever its specific form or level of penetration, clientelism and particularistic social policies are a relatively widespread, legitimate or tolerated component in the workings of welfare states in the extended family of Mediterranean nations and distinguishes these nations from other welfare states. The continuing existence of clientelism in a rapidly changing labor market and welfare state system, and the fact that it has overcome conscious reform efforts specifically intended to eradicate it in many of these countries, are telling. It would appear that clientelism in Mediterranean welfare states can be linked to powerful historical commonalities, particularly those that are related to the process of political mobilization and the establishment of welfare state institutions in these nations. In these contexts, it remains a useful tool with which to deal with the needs of both clients and decision-makers and to facilitate effective efforts to address them.

Conclusion

This chapter has adopted, what can be perhaps described as, a soft welfare state regime approach in its effort to make a case for the existence and analytical usefulness of an extended family of Mediterranean welfare states. In doing so, it acknowledges the critique of the employment of welfare state regime typologies but, at the same time, assumes that this approach to understanding the dynamics of welfare states is a useful way in which to employ comparative analysis.

Drawing upon existing literature on the Southern European welfare state model and on additional welfare states in the Mediterranean, the claim here has been for the inclusion of additional welfare states into, what has been described as, an extended family of Mediterranean welfare states. Thus, it suggests including Cyprus, Israel, Malta, and Turkey in addition to Greece, Italy, Portugal, and Spain, in the analysis.

Undoubtedly the eight nations included in this family of nations differ in various ways, not least in that some have been influenced by the Bismarckian approach while others by a more Beveridgian approach. So while Beveridge and Bismarck evidently did not take a Mediterranean cruise together, their spirits certainly did appear to spend time in all of these nations. As such, some of the features typically associated with the Southern European Model, such as an emphasis on contributions and marked duality in welfare provision, are not necessarily common to all the nations discussed here. However, despite the differences between these nations, it would appear that apart from their geographic proximity to the Mediterranean Sea, they have other significant characteristics in common. A common modern history of late industrialization, authoritarian or colonial rule, and ongoing threats to the stability and efficiency of the state have contributed to similarities in the structuring of their welfare states and in their ability to achieve acceptable welfare outcomes. Moreover this chapter has focused upon the impact of religion, the role of the family, and the existence of various forms of clientelistic relationships in the political arena in order to underscore some additional core features that indicate that these nations may indeed constitute a family of welfare states that has distinctive characteristics. As a consequence of these common features, we find that these nations are generally characterized by less resources, relatively low levels of social expenditure, weak state support for the poor, a major role for the family and religious organizations in the provision of welfare, relatively low levels of labor market participation (particularly among women), and overall limited success in alleviating poverty and overcoming social and economic gaps.

This chapter comprises a very initial attempt to sketch the contours of an extended family of welfare states and can do little more than offer direction for future research and identify interesting avenues for further discussion. Hopefully, this overview of commonalities and differences and the attempt to identify three themes that were crucial to the emergence process of welfare states in these nations and are still evident today, can serve as a basis for more fruitful comparative cross-national research on these welfare states and a better understanding of developments in them. In particular, it can serve as a means to examine issues that are currently on the agenda of policy-makers, civil society, and scholars in these nations. These will clearly include issues such as gender and children, immigration, care for the elderly, and transformation within the labor market.

Acknowledgments I would like to gratefully acknowledge the assistance of Michal Alfasi in the collection of data for this paper and that of David Levi-Faur for his very useful comments.

References

Aassve, A., Mazzuco, S., & Mencarini, L. (2005). Childbearing and wellbeing: A comparative analysis of European welfare regimes. *Journal of European Social Policy, 15*(4), 283–299.

Ajzenstadt, M., & Gal, J. (2001). Appearances can be deceptive: Gender in the Israeli welfare state. *Social Politics, 8*, 292–324.

Akalin, A. (2007). Hired as a caregiver, demanded as a housewife. *European Journal of Women's Studies, 14*(3), 209–225.

Alber, J. (1986). Germany. In P. Fora (Ed.), *Growth to limits, V.II* (pp. 1–154). Berlin: Walter de Gruyter.

Algun, Y., & Cahuc, P. (2006). Job protection: The macho hypothesis. *Oxford Review of Economic Policy*, *22*(3), 390–410.

Andreotti, A., Garcia, S. M., Gomez, A., Hespanha, P., Kazepov, Y., & Mingione, E. (2001). Does a Southern European model exist? *Journal of European Area Studies*, *9*(1), 43–62.

Arnstein, A., Mazzuco, S., & Mencarini, L. (2005). Childbearing and well-being: A comparative analysis of European welfare regimes. *Journal of European Social Policy*, *15*(4), 283–299.

Arts, W., & Gellisen, J. (2002). Three worlds of welfare capitalism or more? *Journal of European Social Policy*, *12*(2), 137–158.

Bambra, C. (2005). Cash versus services: Worlds of welfare' and the decommodification of cash benefits and health care services. *Journal of Social Policy*, *34*(2), 195–213.

Bambra, C. (2006). Research note: Decommodification and the worlds of welfare revisited. *Journal of European Social Policy*, *16*(1), 73–80.

Bambra, C. (2007). A two-dimensional discriminate analysis of welfare state regime theory. *Social Policy and Administration*, *41*(1), 1–28.

Bonoli, G. (1997). Classifying welfare states: A two-dimensional approach. *Journal of Social Policy*, *26*(3), 351–372.

Buğra, A. (2007). Poverty and citizenship: An overview of the social policy environment in Republican Turkey. *International Journal of Middle East Studies*, *39*, 33–52.

Buğra, A., & Keyder, C. (2006). The Turkish welfare regime in transformation. *Journal of European Social Policy*, *16*(3), 211–228.

Castles, F. C. (1993). Introduction. In F. G. Castles (Ed.), *Families of nations* (pp. xiii–xxiii). Aldershot: Dartmouth.

Castles, F. G. (1994). On religion and public policy: Does Catholicism make a difference? *European Journal of Political Research*, *25*, 19–40.

Castles, F. G. (1995). Welfare state development in Southern Europe. *West European Politics*, *18*(2), 291–313.

Castles, F. G. (2004). *The future of the welfare state*. Oxford: Oxford University Press.

Charbit, M. (2003). Shas between identity construction and clientelistic dynamics: The creation of an 'identity clientelism'. *Nationalism and Ethnic Politics*, *9*(3), 102–128.

Chesnais, J. C. (1996). Fertility, family, and social policy in contemporary Western Europe. *Population and Development Review*, *22*(4), 729–739.

Clasen, J., & Siegel, N. A. (2007). *Investigating welfare state change: The 'dependent variable problem' in comparative analysis*. Cheltenham, UK: Edward Elgar.

Cnaan, R. A., & Boddie, S. C. (2002). *The invisible caring hand: American congregations and the provision of welfare*. New York: New York University Press.

Cousins, M. (2005). *European welfare states*. London: Sage.

Da Roit, B. (2007). Changing intergenerational solidarities within families in a Mediterranean welfare state. *Current Sociology*, *55*(2), 251–269.

Danopolous, C. P. (2004). Religion, civil society, and democracy in Orthodox Greece. *Journal of Southern Europe and the Balkans*, *6*(1), 41–55.

Davaki, K., & Mossialos, E. (2005). Plus ça change: Health sector reform in Greece. *Journal of Health Politics, Policy and Law*, *30*(1–2), 143–167.

Dean, H., & Khan, Z. (1997). Muslim perspectives on welfare. *Journal of Social Policy*, *26*(2), 193–210.

Doron, A. (1994). The effectiveness of the Beveridge model at different stages of socio-economic development: The Israeli experience. In J. Hills, J. Ditch, & H. Glennerster (Eds.), *Beveridge and social security* (pp. 189–202). Oxford: Oxford University Press.

Doron, A. (2001). Social welfare policy in Israel: Developments in the 1980s and 1990s. *Israel Affairs*, *7*(4), 153–180.

Doron, A. (2003). The Israeli welfare regime: Changes and their social implications. *Israeli Sociology*, *5*(2), 417–434 (Hebrew).

Eikemo, T. A., Bambra, C., Judge, K., & Ringdal, K. (2008). Welfare state regimes and self-perceived health in Europe: A multilevel analysis. *Social Science and Medicine, 66*(11), 2281–2295.

Eisenstadt, S. N., & Roniger, L. (1984). *Patrons, clients and friends.* Cambridge, UK: Cambridge University Press.

Esping-Andersen, G. (1990). *The three worlds of welfare capitalism.* Cambridge, UK: Polity Press.

Esping-Andersen, G. (1999). *Social foundations of postindustrial economies.* Oxford: Oxford University Press.

European Commission. (2006). *Euro-Mediterranean statistics.* Luxembourg: European Union.

Eurostat. (2007). *Social protection in the European Union.* Luxembourg: European Union.

Falzon, M.-A. (2007). God protect me from my friends: Prelates, politicians and social welfare in contemporary Malta. *Journal of Mediterranean Studies, 17*(1), 47 – 72.

Fargion, V. (1997). Social assistance and the North–South cleavage in Italy. In M. Rhodes (Ed.), *Southern European welfare states: Between crisis and reform* (pp. 135–154). London: Frank Cass.

Featherstone, K. (2005). Introduction: "Modernization" and the structural constraints of Greek politics. *West European Politics, 28*(2), 223–241.

Ferreira, L. V. (2008). Persistent poverty: Portugal and the Southern European welfare regime. *European Societies, 10*(1), 49–71.

Ferrera, M. (1996). The 'Southern Model' of welfare in Social Europe, *Journal of European Social Policy, 6*(1), 17–37.

Ferrera, M. (2008). The European welfare state: Golden achievements, silver prospects. *West European Politics, 31*(1–2), 82–107.

Ferrera, M., Hemerijick, A., & Rhodes, M. (2001). Recasting European welfare states for the 21st century. In S. Leibfried (Ed.), *Welfare state futures* (pp. 151–170). Cambridge, UK: Cambridge University Press.

Fouarge, D., & Layte, R. (2005). Welfare regimes and poverty dynamics: The duration and recurrence of poverty spells in Europe. *Journal of Social Policy, 34*(3), 407–426.

Gal, J. (2004). Decommodification and beyond: A comparative analysis of work injury programs. *Journal of European Social Policy, 14,* 55-69.

Ginn, J., & Fast, J. (2006). Employment and social integration in midlife. *Research on Aging, 28*(6), 669–690.

Gough, I. (1996). Social assistance in Southern Europe. *South European Society and Politics, 1*(1), 1–23.

Gough, I., & Wood, G. (2004). *Insecurity and welfare regimes in Asia, Africa and Latin America.* Cambridge, UK: Cambridge University Press.

Grasselli, P., Montesi, C., & Iannone, P. (2006). *Mediterranean models of welfare towards families and children.* Paper presented at the 46th Congress of the European Regional Science Association, Perugia, Italy.

Greeley, A. (1989). Protestant and Catholic: Is the analogical imagination extinct? *American Sociological Review, 54*(4), 485–502.

Guerrero, T. J., & Naldini, M. (1997). Is the south so different? Italian and Spanish families in comparative perspective. In M. Rhodes (Ed.), *Southern European welfare states: Between crisis and reform* (pp. 42–66). London: Frank Cass.

Guibentif, P. (1997). The transformation of the Portuguese social security system. In M. Rhodes (Ed.), *Southern European welfare states: Between crisis and reform* (pp. 219–239). London: Frank Cass.

Guiliano, P. (2007). Living arrangements in Western Europe: Does cultural origin matter? *Journal of the European Economic Association, 5*(5), 927–952.

Guillén, A. M., & Alvarez, S. (2004). The EUs impact on the Spanish welfare state: The role of cognitive Europeanization. *Journal of European Social Policy, 14*(3), 285–299.

Guillén, A. M., Álvarez, S., & Adão e Silva, P. (2003). Redesigning the Spanish and Portuguese welfare states: The impact of accession in the European Union. *South European Society and Politics, 8*(1–2), 231–268.

Heidenheimer, A. J. (1983). Secularization patterns and the westward spread of the welfare state, 1883–1983. *Comparative Social Research, 6,* 3–65.

Heper, M. (2002). Conclusion – The consolidation of democracy versus democratization in Turkey. *Turkish Studies, 3*(1), 138–146.

Hill, J., Ditch, J., & Glennerster, H. (eds.). (1994). Beveridge and social security: An international Perspective Oxford: Oxford University Press.

Hopkin, J. (2001). A 'southern model' of electoral mobilization? Clientelism and electoral politics in Spain. *West European Politics, 24*(1), 115–136.

Hopkin, J., & Mastropaolo, A. (2001). From patronage to clientelism: Comparing the Italian and Spanish experiences. In S. Piattoni (Ed.), *Clientelism, interests and democratic representation* (pp. 152–171). Cambridge: Cambridge University Press.

Huber, E., & Stephens, J. D. (2001). *Development and crisis of the welfare state.* Chicago: University of Chicago Press.

Hudson, R., & Lewis, J. R. (1984). Capital accumulation: The industrialization of southern Europe? In A. M. Williams (Ed.), *Southern Europe transformed* (pp. 179–207). London: Harper & Row.

Işik, O., & Pinarcioglu, M. M. (2006). Geographies of a silent transition: A geographically weighted regression approach to regional fertility differences in Turkey. *European Journal of Population, 22,* 399–421.

Jaffe, E. D. (1992). Sociological and religious origins of the non-profit sector in Israel. *International Sociology, 8*(2), 159–176.

Jensen, C. (2008). Worlds of welfare services and transfers. *Journal of European Social Policy, 18*(2), 151–162.

Kahl, S. (2005). The religious roots of modern poverty policy: Catholic, Lutheran, and Reformed Protestant traditions compared. *European Journal of Sociology, 46,* 91–126.

Kasza, G. J. (2002). The illusion of welfare 'regimes'. *Journal of Social Policy, 31*(2), 271–287.

Kiliç, A. (2008). The gender dimensions of social policy reform in Turkey: Towards equal citizenship? *Social Policy and Administration, 42*(5), 487–503.

Kleinman, M. (2002). *A European welfare state?* Houndmills: Palgrave.

Kuran, T. (2003). Islamic redistribution through *Zakat.* In M. Bonner, M. Ener, & A. Singer (Eds.), *Poverty and charity in Middle Eastern contexts* (pp. 275–293). Albany: State University of New York Press.

Kvist, J., & Saari, L. (Eds.) (2007). *The Europeanisation of social protection.* Bristol: Policy Press.

Lewis, J. (1997). Gender and welfare regimes. Further thoughts. *Social Politics, 4,* 160 – 177.

Liebfried, S. (1992). Towards a European welfare state? On integrating poverty regimes into the European community. In Z. Ferge & J. Kolberg (Eds.), *Social policy in a changing Europe* (pp. 245–279). Vienna: Campus.

Mabbet, D., & Bolderson, H. (1999). Theories and methods in comparative social policy. In J. Clasen (Ed.), *Comparative social policy* (pp. 34–56). Oxford: Blackwell.

Mâitre, B., Nolan, B., & Whelan, C. T. (2005). Welfare regimes and household income packages in the European Union. *Journal of European Social Policy, 15*(2), 157–171.

Makrides, V. N., & Molokotos-Liederman, L. (2004). Introduction. *Social Compass, 51*(4), 459–470.

Manning, N. (2007). Turkey, the EU and social policy. *Social Policy and Society, 6*(4), 491–502.

Manow, P. (2004). *'The good, the bad, and the ugly' – Esping-Andersen's regime typology and the religious roots of the Western welfare state.* MPIfG Working Paper 04/3, September 2004.

Manow, P., & van Kersbergen, K. (2006). *The impact of class coalitions, cleavage structures and church-state conflicts on welfare state development.* Working Papers Political Science No. 2006/03, Department of Political Science, Vrije Universiteit Amsterdam.

Manski, C. F., & Meyshar, J. (2002). *Private and social incentives for fertility: Israeli puzzles.* Working Paper 8984. Cambridge, MA: NBER.

Martin, C. (1997). Social welfare and the family in Southern Europe. In M. Rhodes (Ed.), *Southern European welfare states: Between crisis and reform* (pp. 23–41). London: Frank Cass.

Matsaganis, M., Ferrera, M., Capucha, L., & Moreno, L. (2003). Mending nets in the South: Anti-poverty policies in Greece, Italy, Portugal and Spain. *Social Policy and Administration*, *37*(1), 639–655.

Mitchell, J. P. (2002). Corruption and clientelism in a 'systemless system': The Europeanization of Maltese political culture. *Southern European Society & Politics*, *7*(1), 43–62.

Moreno, L. (2002). *Mediterranean welfare and 'Superwomen'*. Madrid: Unidad de Políticas Comparadas.

Moreno, L. (2004). Spain's transition to new risks: A farewell to 'Superwomen'? In P. Taylor-Gooby (Ed.), *New risks, new welfare* (pp. 133–156). Oxford: Oxford University Press.

Moreno, L. (2006). *The model of social protection in Southern Europe: Enduring characteristics?* Madrid: Unidad de Políticas Comparadas.

Morlino, J. (2002). The Europeanisation of Southern Europe. In A. C. Pinto & N. S. Teixeira (Eds.), *Southern Europe and the making of the European Union, 1945–1980s* (pp. 237–260). Boulder: Social Science Monographs.

Muffels, R., & Fouarge, D. (2004). The role of European welfare states in explaining resources deprivation. *Social Indicators Research*, *68*, 299–330.

Mullard, M., & Pirotta, G. A. (2008). The politics of public expenditure in Malta. *Commonwealth and Comparative Politics*, *46*(1), 128–141.

Naldini, M. (2003). *The family in the Mediterranean welfare states*. London: Frank Cass.

Naldini, M., & Saraceno, C. (2008). Social and family policies in Italy: Not totally frozen but far from structural reforms. *Social Policy and Administration*, *42*(7), 733–748.

OECD. (2007). *The social expenditure database*. Accessed 15 May 2008 from http://www.oecd.org/dataoecd

Ogg, J. (2005). Social exclusion and insecurity among older Europeans: The influence of welfare regimes. *Ageing & Society*, *25*, 69–90.

Okun, B. S., Oliver, A. L., & Khait-Marelly, O. (2007). The public sector, family structure, and labor market behavior – Jewish mothers in Israel. *Work and Occupations*, *34*(2), 174–204.

Opielka, M. (2008). Christian foundations of the welfare state: Strong cultural values in comparative perspective. In W. van Oorschot, M. Opielka, & B. Pfau-Effinger (Eds.), *Culture and welfare state* (pp. 89–114). Cheltenham, UK: Edward Elgar.

Orloff, A. S. (1993). Gender and the social right of citizenship: The comparative analysis of gender relations and welfare states, *American Sociological Review*, *58*, 303 – 328.

Palier, B., & Martin, C. (2007). Editorial introduction – From 'a frozen landscape' to structural reform: The sequential transformation of Bismarckian welfare systems. *Social Policy and Administration*, *41*(6), 535–554.

Piattoni, S. (2001). *Clientelism, interests, and democratic representation*. Cambridge, UK: Cambridge University Press.

Prince Cook, L. (2009). Gender equity and fertility in Spain and Italy. *Journal of Social Policy*, *38*(1), 123–140.

Requena, M. (2005). The secularization of Spanish society: Change in religious practice. *Southern European Society and Politics*, *10*(3), 369–390.

Rhodes, M. (1997). Southern European welfare states: Identity, problems and prospects for reform. In M. Rhodes (Ed.), *Southern European welfare states: Between crisis and reform* (pp. 1–22). London: Frank Cass.

Rocha, J. A. O., & Araújo, J. F. F. E. (2007). Administrative reform in Portugal: Problems and prospects. *International Review of Administrative Sciences*, *73*(4), 583–596.

Roniger, L. (2004). Review: Political clientelism, democracy, and market economy. *Comparative Politics*, *36*(3), 353–375.

Sapelli, G. (1995). *Southern Europe since 1945*. London and New York: Longman.

Saraceno, C. (Ed.) (2002). *Social assistance dynamics in Europe: National and local poverty regimes*. Bristol: The Policy Press.

Scruggs, L., & Allan, J. (2006). Welfare state decommodification in 18 OECD countries: A replication and revision. *Journal of European Social Policy, 16*(1), 55–72.

Shefter, M. (1994). *Political parties and the state.* Princeton, NJ: Princeton University Press.

Shekeris, A. (1998). The Cypriot welfare state: Contradiction and crisis? *The Cyprus Review, 10*(2), 113–134.

Sherwin, B. (2000). *Jewish ethics for the twenty-first century.* Syracuse: Syracuse University Press.

Sotiropoulos, D. A. (2004a). The EUs impact on the Greek welfare state: Europeanization on paper? *Journal of European Social Policy, 14*(3), 267–284.

Sotiropoulos, D. A. (2004b). Southern European public bureaucracies in comparative perspective. *West European Politics, 2*(3), 405–422.

Symeonidou, H. (1997). Social protection in contemporary Greece. In M. Rhodes (Ed.), *Southern European welfare states: Between crisis and reform* (pp. 67–86). London: Frank Cass.

Taylor-Gooby, P. (2002). *Welfare states under pressure.* London: Sage.

Toren, N. (2003). Tradition and transition: Family change in Israel. *Gender Issues, 21*(2), 60–76.

Trifiletti, R. (1999). Southern European welfare regimes and the worsening position of women. *Journal of European Social Policy, 9*(1), 49–64.

Tsakloglou, P., & Papadopolous, F. (2002). Aggregate level and determining factors of social exclusion in 12 European countries. *Journal of European Social Policy, 12*(3), 211–225.

van Kersbergen, K. (1995). *Social capitalism: A study of Christian democracy and the welfare state.* London: Routledge.

van Oorschot, W. (2007). Culture and social policy: A developing field of study. *International Journal of Social Welfare, 16*, 129–139.

Venieris, D. N. (1997). Dimensions of social policy in Greece. In M. Rhodes (Ed.), *Southern European welfare states: Between crisis and reform* (pp. 260–269). London: Frank Cass.

Vogel, J. (2003). The Family. *Social Indicators Research, 64*(3), 373–391.

Weber, M. (1958). *The Protestant ethic and the spirit of capitalism.* New York: Charles Scribner's Sons.

Weingrod, A. (1968). Patrons, patronage and political parties. *Comparative Studies in Society and History, 10*(4), 377–400.

Wilensky, H. (1981). Leftism, catholicism and democratic corporatism: The role of political parties in recent welfare state development. In P. Flora & A. J. Heidenheimer (Eds.), *The development of welfare states in Europe and America* (pp. 345–382). New Brunswick: Transaction.

Williams, A. M. (1984). Introduction. In A. M. Williams (Ed.), *Southern Europe transformed* (pp. 1–32). London: Harper & Row.

Zöllner, D. (1982). Germany. In P. A. Köhler, H. F. Zacher, & M. Partington (Eds.), *The evolution of social insurance, 1880–1980* (pp. 1–92). London: Frances Pinter.

Part III
Country Studies

Children, Gender and Families in the Italian Welfare State

Valeria Fargion

Introduction

Notably, the Italian welfare state suffers from major functional and distributive problems originating from the country's distorted pattern of social spending. In particular, while pension spending is around 15 percentage points above the EU25 average, expenditure for family policies only accounts for 4% of total social spending, compared to an EU average of 8%. Given this data, it is hardly surprising that the major expert on the Italian social protection system, Maurizio Ferrera, devoted his latest book "E' tempo di donne" to this topic. In his opening remarks, the author asserts that Italy is confronted with a vicious circle which is characterized by "too many women at home, too many empty cradles, too many poor children" (Ferrera, 2008, p. 1). The arguments presented by Ferrera complement the rich body of literature by feminist writers, and offer a clear set of policy recommendations aimed at strengthening the labour market position of women and policies attempting to reconcile work–family tensions.

Because of the fact that much has been written regarding Italy's dismal record in gender equity, financial support to families, childcare services and child poverty, one might think there is little more to add (Saraceno, 1998, 2005; Saraceno & Leira, 2008; Nunni & Vezzosi, 2007). This chapter rises to the challenge by addressing three different issues which have received insufficient attention, especially in comparative studies. First, family policies were not always marginalized, as is currently the case, and it is important to understand when, how and why they lost ground. Hence, the first part of the paper presents some preliminary results from a joint research project with Ferrera and Matteo Jessoula undertaken for the Historical Unit of the Bank of Italy. This project aims at shedding light on the origins of the distorted pattern of Italian social spending, and focuses on the 1950s and early 1960s when family allowances still played a major role within the overall social protection system.

V. Fargion (✉)
Department of Political Science and Sociology, University of Florence, Florence, Italy
e-mail: valeria.fargion@unifi.it

M. Ajzenstadt, J. Gal (eds.), *Children, Gender and Families in Mediterranean Welfare States*, Children's Well-Being: Indicators and Research 2, DOI 10.1007/978-90-481-8842-0_5, © Springer Science+Business Media B.V. 2010

While the first part of the paper places current problems into a historical perspective, the next part shows that when addressing children, gender and family issues in the Italian case, one also needs to take into consideration the territorial dimension; particularly the North–South divide. To achieve this purpose, the chapter provides the most recent statistical information on fertility rates, female occupation and child poverty by geographical area, and discusses the impact of migration flows.

Finally, the last section updates available information from existing literature by illustrating the policy measures introduced by the short-lived Prodi Government, and discusses their limitations. The concluding remarks are devoted to considering unresolved issues which the centre-left coalition handed over to the current centre-right majority and addresses the prospects for the future.

The 1950s and 1960s: When Italy Turned from a "Family Friendly" State to a "Pension" State

Studies on Italian family policies always emphasize the role of Fascism in introducing family allowances, and usually connect them to the regime's demographic goals. While in fact, the story is slightly more complicated,[1] historical accounts tend to devote far too little attention to what happened in the 15 years following the collapse of the fascist regime and the return to democracy. This time period is crucial in the long-term perspective because the distorted pattern of Italian social spending originated precisely during those years. Surprisingly, as compared to current figures, Table 1 shows that Italian public expenditure for family benefits was higher than pension spending throughout the first part of the 1950s.

This distribution of social expenditure was in accordance with the profile of social spending which the newly established Republic inherited from the Fascist Regime. In fact, in this policy area, the 1950s witnessed great continuity from the previous period, with only incremental adjustments to the 1940 law on family benefits. The latter had re-arranged pre-existing programs and most importantly introduced a separate administration for family benefits (*Cassa Unica degli Assegni Familiari*) within the major social insurance fund, INPS, which maintained the same financial arrangements until 1960.

Despite the climate of ideological confrontation typical of the 1950s, there was widespread consensus on the nature and function of family benefits. Christian Democrats and Communists agreed on the basic principles underpinning what many years later Lewis and Ostner labelled "the male breadwinner model". The

---

[1] Following Fascist trade unions' pressure, family allowances were originally established to compensate industrial workers with large families for the reductions in working hours which were introduced in the early 1930s in order to create new jobs in a context of mass unemployment. As the economy recovered during the mid-1930s the program was extended to agricultural workers and swiftly linked to the regime's demographic ambitions.

Table 1 Expenditure for income maintenance programs in the private sector, Italy, 1952–1955 (billions of current lira)

Income maintenance programs	Years			
	1952	1953	1954	1955
Pensions	169	198	222	274
Family benefits	209	273	303	323
Unemployment	20	21	19	21
Tuberculosis	34	35	39	42
Sickness benefits	81	96	106	120
Work injuries Industrial sector	27	27	31	36
Work injuries Agricultural sector	3	4	4	5

Source: Camera dei Deputati (1957, various pages)

following statement by the 1957 Parliamentary Inquiry Committee on workers' living conditions is illuminating:

> The traditional wage system causes a number of inequities, in spite of the apparent fairness. Two workers who do the same job for the same firm, and are equally cleaver in doing their work, will receive the same hourly pay and at the end of the week will get the same pay check. However, if the first one, for instance, has to support only his wife, while the other has to support a large number of children, who are too young to work, and perhaps even his disabled parents, there can be little doubt that – in spite of the household heads having exactly the same social, occupational and salary position – the standard of living of the two families will greatly differ, with the larger family suffering from the greatest hardship [...] The combination of wages and family benefits determines in a quite satisfactory way the so called family salary, that is to say that particular wage system which – by considering the different composition of various households – tends to eliminate the abovementioned disadvantages which are produced by a rigid implementation of the general principle of "equal pay for equal work".[2]

Yet, to fully understand what family benefits represented within the Italian social protection system of the 1950s, one needs to consider two specific aspects: the profile of beneficiaries and funding arrangements. Table 11 of the Appendix highlights the fragmentary nature of the scheme by documenting the considerable variation in benefit levels for the eight different occupational categories of employees which the program covered. However, the information provided in the table, particularly what might appear as bizarre differences in the benefit level for different family members among the various occupational sectors, only tells us one part of the story.

To get the full picture, one needs to consider in greater detail which family members were entitled to benefits and the geographical distribution of the relevant expenditure. In contrast to most other countries, family benefits were granted to workers' parents. However, in addition, coverage could be extended to a long list of

---

[2]Camera dei deputati (1957, p. 871).

other relatives. All that was needed was a deed legally signed by the worker stating that he was responsible for supporting his brother, sister, nephew among others. Under these circumstances, it was legally possible for a worker to receive family allowances for as many as 15 to 20 people. This situation allowed for widespread misuse of the program, especially in economically deprived areas. The large number of court cases[3] during those years confirm that fraudulent behaviour on the part of employees, and also on the part of employers, was not rare. Perhaps even more interesting is that politicians and trade union officials openly showed a benevolent attitude towards this state of affairs. By examining cash flows for family benefits in the different parts of the country one can begin to understand why this kind of misuse was not openly condemned. Table 2 addresses this issue by providing 1960 regional data on revenues and spending for family benefits in each of the three main occupational sectors of salaried workers. The evidence presented in the table shows a very remarkable redistribution from the northern to the southern part of the country[4] for the industrial and the trade sector, while agriculture displays a negative balance between social contributions and benefits throughout the country. In the case of Sicily, for instance, benefits are eight times higher than the contributions which were collected in the region that year.

Against this backdrop, one can better appreciate the following statement published in the official journal of the social insurance fund, INPS:

> The current system might enhance fraud attempts, but we should not forget that in fact what is certainly a fraud also achieved the goal of alleviating poverty among the people who have not benefited from the golden rain of the economic miracle or have received only a few drops of it; in many cases it served to guarantee social peace in economically depressed areas; in other cases it granted more humane living conditions to under-occupied categories of workers – in conjunction with a benefit which is inappropriately named agricultural unemployment compensation but is in fact another wage complement. (Masini, 1962, p. 15)

The evidence presented thus far suggests that Italian family benefits did not work exactly in the same way as in other Bismarkian welfare states. While formally part of the social insurance system, family benefits in the Italian case were not granted on the basis of standardized and highly institutionalized procedures. Quite to the contrary, the existing scheme allowed for considerable discretion in identifying beneficiaries – a feature which is typical of public assistance rather than social insurance. This logic and the operational management of family benefits during the 1950s and 1960s reinforces Ferrera's (1996) argument regarding the Southern model of welfare. According to the author, Southern European countries

---

[3]Evidence can be found in the 1950s and 1960s issues of "*La Rivista Italiana di Previdenza Sociale*" which regularly covered Court judgements on the topic and also usually published experts' comments.

[4]The first eight regions listed in Table 2 are in the Northern part of the country; Tuscany, Umbria, the Marches and Latium belong to Central Italy, while the remaining seven regions are in the South (Sardinia is usually included in this latter group). The term *Mezzogiorno* is also used when referring to Southern regions and the two major islands Sicily and Sardinia.

Table 2 Social contributions and family benefits in the industrial, trade and agricultural sector by region (in lira), 1960

Regions	Industry		Trade		Agriculture	
	Social contributions	Family benefits	Social contributions	Family benefits	Social contributions	Family benefits
Piedmont	53,300,007	29,959,037	3,680,782	1,834,735	946,054	990,264
Valle d' Aosta	1,400,342	1,291,983	113,846	62,449	2,478	27,059
Lombardy	111,626,538	70,466,147	12,481,542	7,200,770	2,939,036	5,455,843
Trentino Alto-Adige	4,525,601	4,845,613	1,398,875	841,139	79,172	303,787
Veneto	24,870,349	25,059,989	3,872,769	3,328,799	958,127	2,315,267
Friuli Venezia Giulia	8,144,492	7,160,068	1,551,414	938,582	132,072	234,912
Liguria	19,914,127	15,142,305	2,893,058	1,506,530	67,616	63,987
Emilia Romagna	24,254,521	18,187,571	4,210,965	2,643,462	2,074,124	2,673,869
Tuscany	24,384,197	20,873,713	3,099,333	2,258,151	523,869	877,162
Umbria	3,833,674	3,928,566	389,166	329,357	91,504	311,759
The Marches	4,702,451	5,122,025	713,991	610,410	92,484	194,106
Latium	24,390,186	25,888,932	5,837,232	4,804,045	877,097	1,696,116
Abruzzi and Molise	3,566,168	5,386,082	538,087	647,523	85,980	418,907
Campania	17,779,097	33,526,390	3,356,345	6,671,720	425,722	2,201,825
Apulia	7,395,235	15,703,249	1,744,272	4,134,233	1,470,870	7,662,456
Basilicata	1,511,277	2,866,601	148,963	458,629	163,078	1,053,471
Calabria	4,186,257	9,932,363	759,218	2,078,491	556,176	2,793,983
Sicily	13,492,901	23,770,221	2,941,520	5,552,524	950,148	7,847,590
Sardinia	5,543,939	9,992,786	713,236	984,935	488,550	1,840,443

display a dualistic system of income maintenance: "on the one hand, we find a group of hyper-protected beneficiaries who are included in the citadels of *garantismo*: typically public employees, white collar workers and private wage-earners of medium and large enterprises working on a full contract with job security. [. . .] On the other hand we find large numbers of under-protected workers and citizens, who only (occasionally) draw meagre benefits and may thus find themselves in conditions of severe hardship. Typically irregular workers in weak sectors without job security: small enterprises, traditional services and agriculture". (Ferrera, 1996, p. 20). In Ferrera's view, it is precisely, the weak sectors of the labour market that "have offered a favourable ground for the emergence and expansion of a clientelistic market in which state transfers to supplement inadequate work incomes are exchanged for party support" (Ferrera, 1996, p. 25). This argument specifically refers to invalidity pensions and agricultural unemployment benefits; although in the case of family benefits there is no "real exchange of individual votes for individual benefits", there is plenty of judicial evidence showing the widespread misuse and manipulation of the program under consideration.

Funding arrangements add a further piece to this puzzle. First of all, family benefits were financed on the basis of a strict pay-as-you-go system. In other words, social contributions were adjusted yearly depending on the amount of benefit spending. Given the rising level of expenditure, in the early 1950s contribution rates were increased repeatedly. Whereas in 1952 the rate for the industrial sector was already as high as 22.50, only 4 years later the corresponding figure reached 32.80, compared to 9% for pensions and 6% for sickness insurance. However, due to the existence of a salary cap, the effective weight on labour costs was in fact very different depending on the size of the firm; the impact was heaviest for small firms as they usually paid a salary lower than the 900 lira daily ceiling. Large firms, instead, ended up by paying an effective rate of about 20% of the average worker's salary. Therefore, on the one hand, the funding system was biased in favour of large industrial plants, but on the other hand, the fact that a salary cap only existed for this program and for the temporary unemployment scheme confirms – as I noted above – that family benefits were largely perceived as having a social assistance rather than a social insurance function.

The situation described so far begins to change from the late 1950s and early 1960s onwards. Table 3 provides very clear evidence of the progressive and inexorable decline of family benefits as a proportion of the Italian GDP. The proportion drops from 2.39 in 1960 to 1.66 at the end of the decade, falling even further during the next 20 years and reaching as little as 0.61 of the GDP in 1990. The 1950s and 1960s appear in sharp contrast also in regard to the contribution family benefits provided to household budgets. Whereas at the beginning of the 1960s the average family benefit represented 10% of per capita GDP by the end of the decade the corresponding figure was only 5.3%. Benefit levels were upgraded but not enough to keep pace with the extraordinary economic growth during those years.

This helps introduce the discussion regarding Italy's abandonment of family support in favour of pensions. Family benefits were crucial during a period which was characterized by salary stagnation as a result of extreme weakness on the part of

Table 3 Family benefits as a
% of GDP, Italy 1960–1990

Years	Family benefits	Years	Family benefits
1960	2.39	1976	1.36
1961	2.31	1977	1.02
1962	2.30	1978	0.95
1963	2.14	1979	0.82
1964	2.02	1980	0.83
1965	2.10	1981	1.01
1966	2.08	1982	0.87
1967	1.96	1983	0.83
1968	1.96	1984	0.77
1969	1.66	1985	0.67
1970	1.51	1986	0.56
1971	1.43	1987	0.52
1972	1.29	1988	0.55
1973	1.09	1989	0.66
1974	1.50	1990	0.61
1975	1.66		

Source: Franco (1993, pp. 119–120)

workers' trade unions and leftist parties, following the 1948 electoral defeat. In fact, while the cost of living and gross salaries increased by 9 and 10.9 percent respectively between 1951 and 1954, during the same period family allowances increased by 51%. The downward trend started with the commencement of the Italian economic miracle in 1958 and the simultaneous strengthening of workers' unions. It is possible, that workers' unions promoted a different balance between the relative generosity of family benefits and wage increases, especially considering who was actually benefiting from the existing program. In fact, after 10 years of salary stagnations, the trade unions were able to negotiate substantial salary increases in the contract renewals of 1957–1958 and this trend continued throughout the 1960s.

By considering, on the one hand, the drainage of resources from the rich industrialized northern triangle to the impoverished South of Italy (as documented by Table 2) and, on the other hand, the heavy concentration of trade union membership in the North of the country, the lack of strong action by the unions in favour of family benefits is not surprising. However, especially at a distance, it is evident that in 1961 the development of this policy area could have taken an entirely different path. In that year Amintore Fanfani became Prime Minister and brought into his Cabinet a strong representation of the socially oriented left wing of the Christian Democratic Party. This opened a "political window" for overcoming the chaotic fragmentation of family benefits and the blatant inequities of the funding system. Indeed, the Social Affairs Minister Fiorentino Sullo immediately presented a draft bill to Parliament which, in his words, was supposed to "lead the way to a social security system".[5] The bill, which was passed into law in October 1961, introduced major changes both on the revenue and the spending side. Benefit levels were homogenized; a decision

---

[5] Senato della Repubblica, III Legislatura, seduta 468, p. 21816.

which led first to a strong benefit increase for the agricultural sector. According to the Minister, "all workers should be treated if possible in the same way with respect to sickness and family support: one cannot draw a distinction between a blue-collar worker of Italy's largest industrial firm – FIAT – and a Sicilian farm labourer. In the case of pensions, the goal should be different, because it is not enough to guarantee a minimum to everyone … it is fair and necessary for pensions to be in line with the salary curve at the end of the working life so that the pension is tightly linked to the worker's past activity and productive capacity".[6]

If one turns from political discourse to real policy implications, the upgrading of family benefits in the agricultural sector appears to be a reaction to the massive migration taking place then, from the Southern to the Northern part of the country. But what really triggered the government's action was the need to find a solution to the permanent imbalance in a number of occupational schemes, which started with the agricultural one. Accounting procedures had always been kept rigidly separate for each category. Schemes running a deficit were allowed to borrow money from schemes running a surplus, but had to pay interest on the transaction. In contrast to this cumbersome system, the idea of merging all the schemes into the same fund, and enabling the use of money irrespective of where it came from, proved very appealing. The government managed to change the funding of the system along these lines but was not as successful when it tried to abolish the salary cap altogether in order to eliminate the privileges enjoyed by large firms as compared to small firms. It is most interesting that the final text was the result of a tripartite agreement with the industrial employers' association (Confindustria), CGIL and CISL, which represented leftist and catholic workers respectively. Bargaining led to a substantial decrease in the contribution rate, but a salary cap was maintained until 1964. The cap was increased from 900 to 2,500 lira for the industrial sector, but large firms managed to lose much less than originally envisaged by the government.

Subsequent events demonstrate that the "political window" which allowed the introduction of the 1961 law was quickly closed as Italy moved to the centre-left governments of the 1960s. This might seem paradoxical, but the considerable electoral losses which the Christian Democratic Party and the Socialist Party suffered as a result of their decision to form a governing coalition, which evoked disapproval by part of their electorate, induced both parties to opt for a very cautious approach to policy making. Throughout the 1960s the decision to eliminate the abovementioned salary cap was continuously postponed to the advantage of industrial employers. In addition, trade unions did not openly side in favour of an adequate upgrading of family allowances. This required an increase on the revenue side and therefore implied lifting the salary cap on contribution rates. However, the unions' priorities were shifting increasingly in favour of pensions. Migration to the industrialized Northern regions left the weaker and less organized farm labourers in the South, while the trade unions increased their membership in the Northern part of the country, representing primarily the interests of the core labour force. Within this context, family

---

[6]Ibid, p. 21815.

benefits were increasingly funnelled to the peripheral sectors of the labour force. In accordance, coverage was extended to small farmers and the unemployed, in 1967 and 1968, respectively. The industrial workforce was more interested in upgrading the dramatically low level of pensions, and managed to achieve its goal with the introduction of earnings-related pensions in 1968.

Under these circumstances, in Italy family benefits are a victim of the political dynamics typical of the Southern model. The core sectors of the labour force were able to obtain job security and peaks of generosity for themselves, especially with respect to certain risks, first of all old age, while disregarding the macroscopic gaps existing in the overall system of social protection.

Women, Children, Families and the North–South Divide

The previous section demonstrates the centrality of the territorial dimension, when trying to understand the political dynamics that marginalized family policies in Italy from the 1960s onwards. Almost 50 years later, the Italian territorial dimension is still crucial to fully appreciate the problems concerning children, women and families that central, regional and local levels of government must address (Fargion, 1997). Three different sets of indicators are particularly relevant: fertility rates, female occupation and child poverty.

The Regional Profile of Fertility Rates

Notably, Italy displays the lowest fertility rates in the European Union, along with Spain and the new Central-Eastern member states. This downward trend started in the mid-1960s and was not interrupted until the mid-1990s. However, if we look at the breakdown by geographical area, Fig. 1 shows two different patterns corresponding, on the one hand, to central and northern Italy, and, on the other hand, to Southern Italy. In the South, fertility rates have always been higher than in the rest of the country. However, whereas up until the late 1960s there was as much as one point difference between Southern and Centre-Northern fertility rates, a decade later the distance was much smaller, and the two areas are now converging towards the Italian average value of 1.3. This is the result of a continuing decline in birth rates in the South and of a sudden reversal of this trend in the Centre-North, from the mid-1990s onwards.

By looking at Fig. 2, an even clearer picture is evident. The figure provides data on birth rate variations over the 10 year period 1995–2004 for each of the Italian regions. The evidence shows two opposite trends corresponding to the North–South divide: while the six Southern regions and the two major islands all present negative values, the other 12 Central and Northern regions[7] show exactly the opposite trend with the birth rate in Emilia Romagna increasing by as much as 37%.

---

[7] All the regions to the right of the zero axis are centre-northern regions.

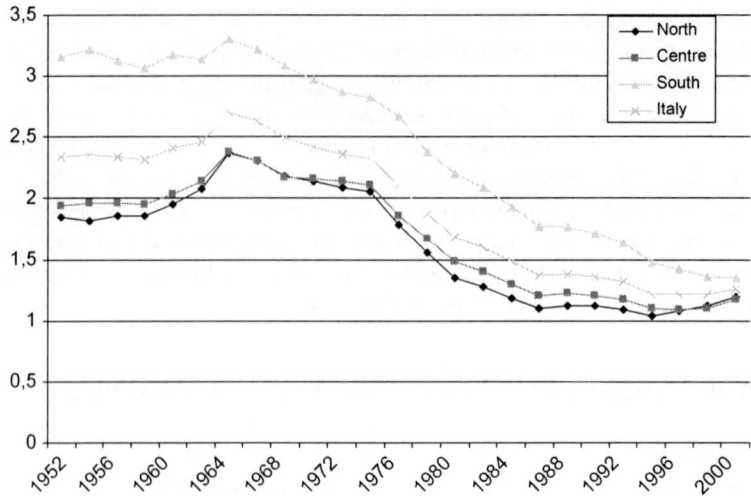

Fig. 1 Italian fertility rates by geographical area, 1952–2001 (Source: ISTAT, 2006b, p. 14)

Immigration is a crucial factor in explaining regional variation in birth rates. According to national statistics, in 2004 resident women with an Italian citizenship had on average 1.26 children, while for immigrant resident women the corresponding figure was twice as much; exactly 2.61, thereby bringing the national average up

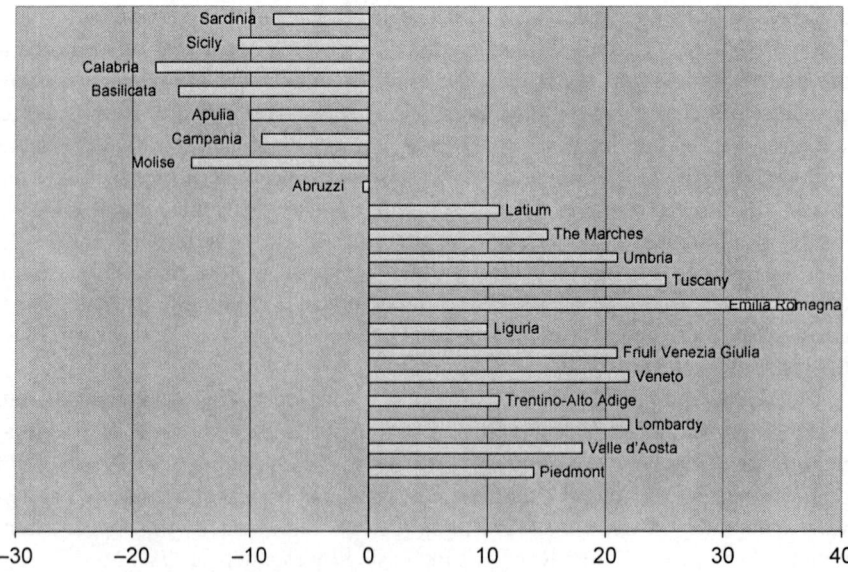

Fig. 2 Percentage of variation in the number of births between 1995 and 2004, by region (Source: ISTAT, 2006a, p. 2)

to 1.33. If we now consider the increase between 1995 (when the number of immigrant resident women was still negligible) and 2004, the data indicates that only half of the increase was due to Italian women, with foreign mothers being responsible for the other 50% of the increase.[8]

Table 4 supports the above argument by providing detailed information on the impact of children with one or both parents of foreign origin on the total number

Table 4 Children with at least one foreign-born parent or both as a % of total resident children born in 1999 and 2004, by Region

Regions	1999		2004	
	At least one foreign-born parent	Both foreign-born parents	At least one foreign-born parent	Both foreign-born parents
Piedmont	8.3	5.5	17.0	12.3
Valle d'Aosta	8.1	4.9	12.1	7.6
Lombardy	9.8	6.9	17.9	14.0
Bolzano-Bozen	6.7	2.9	14.6	8.6
Trento	8.2	5.4	16.1	11.4
Trentino Alto – Adige	7.5	4.1	15.3	10.0
Veneto	8.3	6.0	18.9	15.2
Friuli-Venezia Giulia	6.8	3.5	14.7	9.8
Liguria	6.9	3.5	14.5	9.7
Emilia Romagna	10.1	7.0	19.9	15.3
Tuscany	9.1	5.8	17.3	12.7
Umbria	9.4	6.2	19.4	14.9
The Marches	8.5	5.6	16.6	11.8
Latium	7.2	5.1	12.2	8.3
Abruzzi	4.9	2.4	8.9	5.2
Molise	2.2	0.6	4.7	1.9
Campania	1.6	0.7	3.1	1.5
Apulia	1.6	0.9	3.0	1.9
Basilicata	1.4	0.7	3.1	1.5
Calabria	2.0	0.8	4.0	1.7
Sicily	2.4	1.7	3.1	2.0
Sardinia	2.2	0.8	3.3	1.3
North-west	9.1	6.2	17.4	13.2
North-east	8.7	5.9	18.5	14.2
Centre	8.0	5.5	14.8	10.5
South	1.9	0.9	3.7	1.9
Islands	2.3	1.5	3.1	1.9
Italy	6.0	4.0	12.0	8.7

Source: ISTAT (2006a, p. 4)

---

[8] In detail, the fertility rate went from 1.19 in 1995 to 1.33 in 2004. As mentioned in the text, fertility for Italian women was only 1.26 in 2004; hence, Italian women account for half the increase while the other half is due to immigrant women.

of legally registered births in the various Italian regions. First of all, the proportion of children with two foreign parents more than doubled in only 5 years, increasing from 4% in 1999 to 8% in 2004. However, again, Italy displays a different pattern in the Northern versus the Southern part of the country. The phenomenon under consideration is still marginal in the South and the two major islands Sicily and Sardinia, while in the North-East children with both parents holding foreign citizenship increased from 5.9% to as much as 14.2%. Quite clearly this reflects the economic profile of the country and the different timing of migration flows in the various parts of Italy. As compared to Continental Europe, in Italy migration is a more recent phenomenon. In the more dynamic areas it started around the mid-late 1980s, and thus by now a considerable proportion of immigrant workers have settled down to raise a family.

But focusing on the North–South divide is not enough, because migration is far from being evenly distributed across the Central and Northern regions. In 2004 one out of six newborn babies had foreign parents in Emilia Romagna, Veneto, Lombardy and Umbria, whereas the corresponding figure for Tuscany, Piedmont and the Marches was one out of eight. Intra-regional variation appears even more significant. For instance, in the case of Brescia and Mantova the figure is as high as 25% and is just a little lower for Verona (23.8%), while the Tuscan Province of Prato ranks first with 28.8% of children with foreign parents, almost all of which are of Chinese origin.

In short, Italy's future demographic trends are increasingly influenced by its immigrant population. Finally, because Italian women continue to postpone maternity, the result is that in the Centre-North mothers' average age is 31–32, in contrast with an average of 27 for immigrant women.[9] While it is not clear if this is a problem, in addition to the many implications of an ageing society, in social and economic terms, women themselves are not happy with this state of affairs. Survey data documents that women have less children than they would like (see Table 5).

Table 5 Average number of desired children by age of mother, Italy, 2005

Mother's age	Average number of desired children[a]
<25	2.18
25–29	2.18
30–34	2.16
35–39	2.21
40+	2.35
Total	2.19

[a]The number corresponds to already born children plus the number of children that interviewed women wish to have in the future.
Source: ISTAT (2007a, p. 2)

---

[9]Only 11% of the children born in 2004 had a mother less than 25 years of age. One out of four children, instead, had a mother who was more than 34 years old.

Thus far women have been considered in this paper in their traditional role as mothers. Compared to Northern and most Continental European countries, Italian women find it increasingly difficult to perform this function (Bertolini, 2006; Bettio & Plantanega, 2004; Naldini, 2006a,b). The next section discusses female participation in the labour market in order to determine the extent to which women's occupation "interferes" with maternity.

Female Labour Market Participation

It is well known that in Italy, female activity rates are much lower than in most other European countries, except for Spain and Greece. In 2006, Italy had a female activity rate of 46.3%; 11 points below the European average of 57.4. Although the country as a whole did not meet the 2005 Lisbon target of 57%, by disaggregating the data by geographical area, one can notice immediately that Northern regions actually came very close to the target. Table 6 provides the relevant information, but also sheds light on the different pace in the development of female labour market participation in Centre-North Italy as opposed to the South. The evidence shows that between 1993 and 2004, female activity increased by 10 percentage points in the Central and Northern regions, but only by three points in Southern regions.

This section discusses the extent to which Italian women manage to reconcile family and working life. Unfortunately, the evidence is quite depressing. Marriage or cohabitation does not seem to entail a redistribution of caring responsibilities. Quite the contrary, it apparently overburdens women, pushing them to leave their job more than in the case of single mothers (Bimbi & Trifiletti, 2006). The information provided in Table 7 is intriguing but unequivocal. For married or cohabiting women between the ages of 25–34, the activity rate drops from 78.9 to 60.9 following

Table 6 Activity rates (15–64), by sex and geographical area, Italy 1993–2004

Year	North		Centre		South and islands		Italy	
	Male	Female	Male	Female	Male	Female	Male	Female
1993	71.6	45.3	69.3	39.2	63.8	27.1	68.4	37.7
1994	70.6	45.3	67.8	38.8	61.8	26.4	66.9	37.4
1995	70.6	45.8	66.9	39.3	60.4	25.7	66.2	37.4
1996	70.8	40.0	66.9	40.3	60.1	25.7	66.2	38.2
1997	70.6	47.7	66.8	40.5	59.9	25.9	66.1	38.5
1998	71.1	48.6	67.0	41.5	60.5	26.8	66.5	39.4
1999	71.9	50.1	67.6	43.0	60.5	26.9	67.0	40.4
2000	72.7	51.9	68.3	44.8	61.3	27.5	67.8	41.8
2001	73.2	53.5	68.8	46.5	62.2	29.0	68.4	43.4
2002	73.6	54.5	69.7	47.5	63.0	30.0	69.0	44.4
2003	74.7	55.7	71.3	48.7	63.4	29.9	70.0	45.1
2004	75.0	54.9	71.9	50.2	61.8	30.7	69.7	45.2

Source: Battistoni (2005, p. 23; http://bancadati.italialavoro.it)

Table 7 Female activity rates (25–44) depending on the number and age of children, by status, 2004

Age		Single	Married or cohabiting
25–34	No children	74.3	78.9
	1 child	79.3	60.9
	2 children	62.8	46.3
	More than 2 children	70.4	32.4
	Children aged 0–1	73.8	51.5
	Children aged 0–3	76.4	53.1
	Children aged 0–6	75.9	52.8
35–44	No children	81.9	77.1
	1 child	82.8	70.5
	2 children	80.9	58.9
	More than 2 children	49.3	42.6
	Children aged 0–1	75.5	58.3
	Children aged 0–3	76.8	62.3
	Children aged 0–6	79.6	62.0

Source: Battistoni (2005, p. 39; http://bancadati.italialavoro.it)

the birth of the first child. This is in contrast to the activity rate of 79.3 for single mothers. In the case of two children, activity rates decrease for both categories, but once more women who have a husband or a companion fare much worse: only 46% manage to keep a job, compared to 62.8 of single mothers. Although average figures are higher, a largely similar trend is evident for women in the age group 35–44. Not surprisingly, the younger the children, the lower the activity rate.

As a result of Italy's dismal fertility record, and in an attempt to try to better understand both what prevents mothers from having a second child, and the work–family reconciliation strategies undertaken by working mothers, in 2003 the National Institute for Statistics undertook a sample survey of 50,000 new mothers (Lo Conte, Prati, & Talucci, 2003). The interviews were carried out 18–21 months after childbirth, a point in time at which mothers usually ponder whether or not to have another child. Moreover, this corresponds to the most critical period in terms of work–family reconciliation. The study contains an abundance of information, two of which will be the focus here. According to survey data, 20% of the mothers who had a job when they were pregnant left the labour market by the time of the interview. However, the situation was in fact much worse in the South. Figure 3 illustrates that as many as 30% of the relevant group of mothers was no longer active after the birth of the first child, in contrast to 18% in the Centre-North. Alternatively phrased, in Southern regions the female labour force participation rate is only 30% but as soon as a first child is born the figure drops even further. These two parts of the country display the same behavioural pattern only in the case of women with tertiary education (see Fig. 4). This is a striking exception to what we have seen so far, which suggests that rising female educational levels, albeit not immediately, will help bridge the gap between North and South. Figure 4 shows that as one moves from primary to university-level education, the proportion of Southern women opting for family life in case of maternity drops from over 40% to less than 11%.

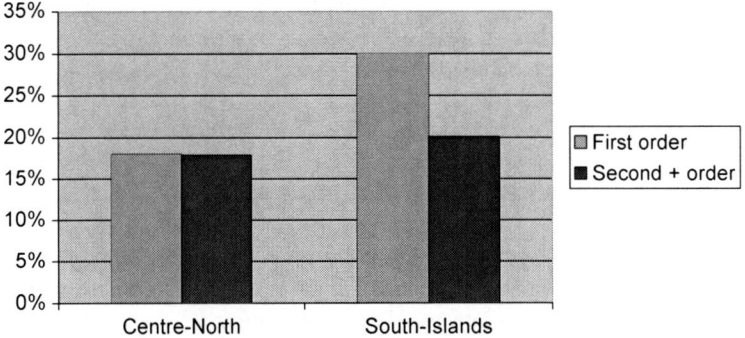

Fig. 3 Mothers leaving the labour market after the birth of the first or the second child, by geographical area (%, 2003 ISTAT sample survey data) (Source: ISTAT, Lo Conte & Prati, 2003, p. 8)

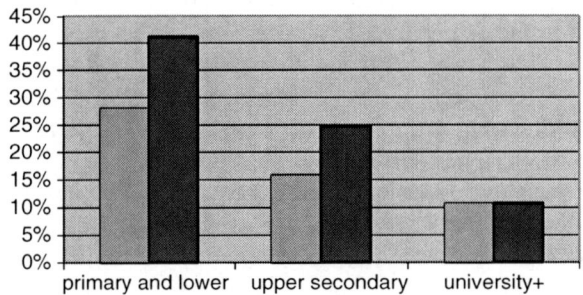

Fig. 4 Mothers leaving or losing the job by geographical area and educational attainment (%, ISTAT, 2003 sample survey data) (Source: ISTAT, Lo Conte & Prati, 2003, p. 10)

The above mentioned survey provides a second piece of information which is highly indicative of an Italian peculiarity in terms of family–work reconciliation strategies. It demonstrates that grandparents play a crucial role in care arrangements for very young children of working mothers. Survey data shows that grandparents take care of 54% of children, in contrast to only 22.4% attending public and private childcare facilities and 11% under the care of a baby-sitter. This state of affairs reflects a complex mix of cultural idiosyncrasies and inadequate public supply of childcare.[10] Little can be done in the short run with respect to the first problem because changing deep-rooted feelings of trust is a long-term process. However, the

---

[10] According to the latest ISTAT data, in the Centre-North childcare services only cover 15.5% of children under three, but the equivalent figure is even much lower in the South: in this area only 4.2% of children have access to public childcare. Considerable variation also exists in both parts of the country: Emilia Romagna ranks first among Centre-Northern regions with a coverage of 27.5, while in the South Campania is at the very bottom with as little as 1.5%. I shall return to this issue in the final section.

government could certainly take responsibility for increasing the number and territorial distribution of childcare facilities. However, before turning to policy responses, child poverty needs to be examined in order to gain the full picture of family welfare in Italy.

The Territorial Dimension of Child Poverty

In January 2008, the EU Social Protection Committee and DG Employment, Social Affairs and Equal Opportunities released a joint report on *Child poverty and well-being in the EU* which offers an excellent opportunity to place Italy's record on child poverty in a comparative perspective. Figure 5 is drawn from this authoritative report: the evidence concerning Italy is definitely not encouraging. Italy is plotted on the top right corner of the figure which corresponds to countries with poverty rates above the EU average for both children and the overall population. In short, Italy combines two negative records. What is most worrisome is that Italian children are disproportionately affected by poverty and social exclusion. Portugal and Spain are in a similar position, but only Romania, Latvia and Poland have a record which is clearly worse. Table 8 offers further elements to grasp the Italian profile of child poverty with respect to the EU. What is perhaps most striking is the extremely limited impact of social transfers in reducing child poverty risk.

By turning to national statistics, as in the case of fertility rates and female occupation, once more the territorial dimension comes to the forefront (Saraceno & Brandolini, 2008). In Southern Italy, the proportion of families below the poverty

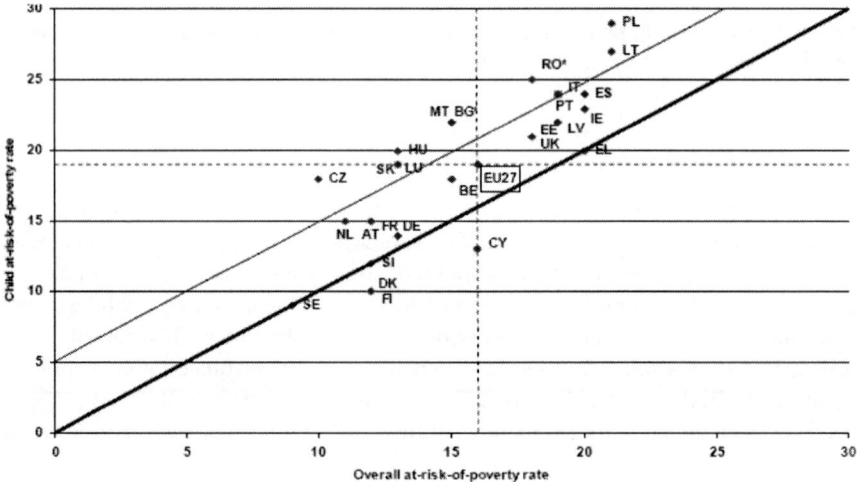

Fig. 5 At-risk-of-poverty in the EU (%) total and children, EU 27 (2005) (Note: The *dotted lines* allow locating countries with poverty rates below/above the EU (weighted) average. The *full lines* indicate how child poverty relates to the overall poverty rate in each country. Child poverty is more than 5 percentage points higher than the overall poverty rate if a country is located above the *thin line*. Source: EU, 2008, p. 14)

Table 8 Main indicators for child poverty, Italy and EU average

Percentage	Child at risk of poverty rate	Child at risk of poverty gap	Children in working poor households	Children in jobless households	Impact of social transfers on child poverty risk
Italy	24	28	18	5.4	23
EU average	19	22	13	9.5	44

Source: EU (2008, p. 103)

line is almost five times higher than in Northern Italy. As a result, as many as 65% of Italian families below the poverty line are concentrated in the Southern part of the country, and the situation is most problematic for large families. Table 9 shows that in 2006 almost one out of two Southern families with three or more children was poor.

A similar disproportion emerges when looking at the typical household of a couple with one child: whereas in the North and in the Centre only 3.9 and 5.4% of families falling in this category was below the poverty line, the corresponding figure for the South was 22%, and goes up to 28% in the case of a couple with two children.

Thus, the picture does not look bright. In spite of the fact that Italy belongs to the G8 and hence to the privileged group of the economically most advanced countries, when it comes to the social needs of women and children the record is certainly not as positive. Social expenditure trends over the last four decades and available studies amply document that policies aimed at addressing the needs of women, children and families have been absolutely marginal in the Italian context, and in line with similar developments in the other Southern European welfare states.

In fact, Chiara Saraceno openly stated a few years ago that in the case of Italy one could detect an explicit family policy only starting with the 1996 Prodi government, even if this still did not correspond to a fully coherent strategy. It has been previously argued (Fargion, 2004) that the Olive Tree coalition, in power from

Table 9 Poor families with children as a % of total families, by family size and geographical area, Italy 2005–2006

Families with children <18	North		Centre		South		Italy	
	2005	2006	2005	2006	2005	2006	2005	2006
With one child	4.8	3.9	5.4	5.4	19.6	22.0	10.1	10.3
With two children	7.2	8.4	8.7	10.6	29.9	28.7	17.2	17.2
With three or more children	_a	8.2	_a	_a	42.7	48.9	27.8	30.2
With at least one child <18	6.3	5.7	7.3	8.3	26.1	27.3	14.1	14.4

[a]Statistically non-reliable data because of the insufficient size of the sample.
Source: ISTAT (2007b, p. 4)

1996 to 2001, continued the reform process initiated by the "technocratic" Cabinets of the 1992–1995 period by focussing on the traditionally marginal policy areas of social care services, family policies and equal opportunities, and attempted to redress entrenched unbalances. At a distance, and especially in the light of the evidence presented in this chapter, it emerges as if Italy was not successful in this endeavour, at least not as much as was hoped in the mid-1990s. But considering the fact that Prodi had a second chance as a result of his electoral victory in 2006, the factors that prevented him from pursuing the policies initiated during his first Cabinet with greater vigour, must be examined.

Family Friendly Policies and the Italian "Pension Trap"

Prodi returned to power following 5 years of centre-right rule. In spite of the rhetoric, the Berlusconi government – in office from 2001 to 2006 – delivered very little with respect to family policies and left a poisoned gift to the new majority in the pension field. In 2004, the so-called Maroni Reform, cut back on seniority benefits, which notably represented one of the major anomalies of the Italian welfare state.[11] The reform fixed a 60 years age threshold, and in an effort to avoid excessive opposition it postponed the requirement to January 2008; beyond Berlusconi's term of office. From 2004 until the end of 2007 (i.e. just prior to the deadline for enforcing the new age threshold) this remained one of the most controversial issues, not only between the centre-right and centre-left coalitions, but also within the latter coalition. Over the first year and a half of Prodi's second Cabinet, this problem monopolized the entire social policy debate to the detriment of any serious discussion on new social needs related to atypical work, youth unemployment, the frail elderly, social exclusion or child poverty. In short, precisely as 5 years earlier, the divide between old and new social risks surfaced again, and the social policy responses showed a similar bias in favour of old risks. Although, according to official estimates, only about 600,000 workers would suffer from the restrictive rules, the three labour confederations and the Re-founded Communist Party adamantly supported their claims and ended up securing 10 billion euro to cover the cost of setting back the age threshold from 60 to 58 years old. Needless to say, this runs counter to all EU policy orientations. While, the trade unions repeatedly underscored that funding would primarily come from savings and streamlining in the management of social insurance funds, the fact remains that this considerable amount of money was not allocated for family support or to combat child poverty.

---

[11] Seniority benefits were originally linked only to the number of insurance years (35 and 20 years for the private and the public sector, respectively) and were payable before the legal retirement age. During the 1990s, the rules were repeatedly tightened by increasing the age threshold. In 1996–1997, in order to be entitled to a seniority pension a private sector employee with a 35 years' contribution record had to be at least 52 years old; in 1998 the age requirement was increased to 54, and in the following 3 years it was increased further, first to 55, then to 56 and finally to 57.

For the first time in Italian post-war history the government included a Minister for the Family, but this, evidently, was not enough to redress the power imbalance between the traditionally well-organized pension constituency and supporters of "women and family friendly" policies. The post was assigned to Rosy Bindi, a highly visible political figure who showed great courage and determination in her capacity as Health Minister during the first Prodi Cabinet.

Bindi initiated a number of policy measures in addition to the government's overall results. Her greatest achievement is probably the 3 year special plan for expanding childcare services. Currently, available childcare facilities cover only 11% of the relevant age group and are distributed unevenly across the country, reaching Nordic levels of coverage only in Emilia Romagna. Figure 6 offers a clear picture of the huge variation existing between North and South by showing that coverage levels drop to as little as 2%, or even less in the cases of Campania and Calabria. The figure also highlights the target set for Southern regions by the 2007–2013 National Strategic Reference Framework for the allocation of EU structural funds. Against this backdrop one can appreciate the government's effort. The budgetary laws of 2007 and 2008 allocated a total of 770 million euro between 2007 and 2009 to create 40,000 new places for children in the 0–2 age group, and a further 24,000 places for the 2–3 age group. Yet, this target remains far below the centre-left electoral commitment to guarantee 100,000 new places. Furthermore, for the near future, the Barcelona target of 33% coverage remains out of reach.

The budgetary law of 2008 also introduced an annual tax rebate up to 632€ to help cover the cost of using public or private childcare facilities. This is despite the fact that the average monthly cost of childcare is 400€, with some municipalities charging more then 500€ (Cittadinanzattiva, 2007).[12] This tax rebate remains a

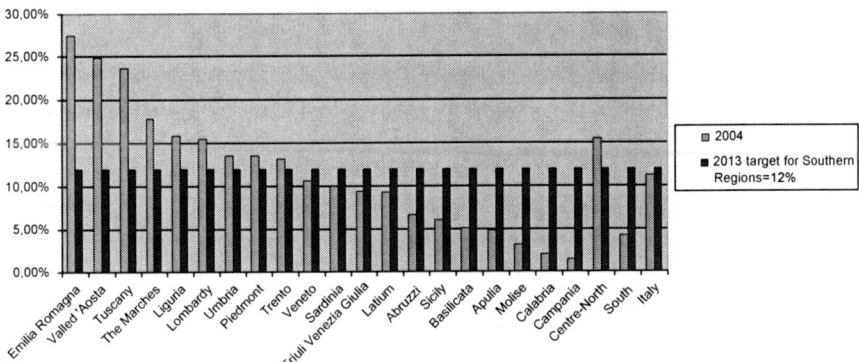

Fig. 6 Coverage of childcare services by Region for 2004, and the 2013 target according to the 2007–2013 National Strategic Reference Framework

---

[12] According to information provided by the website www.cittdinanzaattiva.it, Rome displays the lowest charges with only 146€ per month, while the highest is the case of Lecco at 572€ per month.

mere drop in the ocean, as in the case of the tax rebate for young adults who leave their parents home. As in the case of Spain, young Italians "face great difficulties in forming a couple and establishing an independent household. [...] The progressive delay in the age of marriage or cohabitation reduces the time horizon for achieving the desired fertility. The late emancipation of young Italians is commonly explained by reference to the concomitant failure of the housing market and the high level of temporary employment among young people. The prices for buying a house have more than tripled in the last 15 years [...] and the public renting system is almost non-existent, while the private renting sector offers few alternatives because of its very high prices".[13]

Within this context, the measure which the government introduced was blatantly inadequate. This fact also applies to upgrading family benefits. Some improvements were introduced, particularly for families with disabled dependents, but these remain within the entrenched tradition of piecemeal adjustments. A comprehensive policy is needed. The existing system of child benefits and tax allowances is not only fragmentary, where family allowances are only available for low income public and private employees or families below the poverty line with more than three children, but also produces perverse effects. Experts have pointed out, for instance, that the current tax system favours female inactivity traps in low income families. Yet, the introduction of a universal child benefit or a comprehensive re-organization of child benefit and tax allowances remains out of sight. The list of incremental adjustments is in fact much longer: maternity benefits have been extended to atypical workers, 40 million euro have been allocated to experiment with flexible working time arrangements and money has been allocated to reduce service charges for water, gas and electricity in the case of families with more than four children. These measures certainly represent a step forward, but fall short of re-orienting the Italian social protection system in favour of younger generations, and women and children in particular.

The return to a centre-right government in May 2008 does not seem to enhance a re-orientation of this kind: the discourse is different but the change appears political rhetoric. Only a few months after winning the elections, the Berlusconi Government presented a "Green Book on the Future of the Social Model" which was supposed to outline the overall strategy that the new centre-right majority wants to pursue. The document claims that "the crisis of the Italian social model is primarily a cultural crisis which stems from the fact that the centrality of the person has been overlooked and the role of the family has been repeatedly denied[14]"; the implications of this premise are especially worrisome for social care and long-term care policies, because in the name of prioritising the family there is a risk that public services might be reduced even further, whereas it is precisely the families' capacity to shoulder the caring needs of their dependent members, which so far has counterbalanced the inadequacy of public services. Notably, in the international literature

---

[13]Thus the significant amount of similarities between the Italian and the Spanish case enables the words of a study on Spain by Bernardi (2005) to be applied to Italy.

[14]Ministero del Lavoro, della Salute delle Politiche Sociali (2008, p. 10).

the family is described as the clearing house of the southern welfare model, and what the family needs most badly is to off-load some of its caring burdens, in other words to be concretely supported. But the Government's economic and budgetary plan for 2009–2013 (law 133/2008) seems to go exactly in the opposite direction. First, it cuts down personnel in primary, secondary and higher education considerably; second, it does not contain spending commitments concerning the National Long-term Care Fund established by the previous centre-left cabinet.[15] Both decisions will have a negative impact on families by reducing the quantity and quality of educational and social care services. In detail, over the period 2009–2012 the total number of teachers will be cut by 10.37% – which corresponds to a decrease of 87,400 positions: it is hard to believe that this will not result in a reduction of day school hours, as the Education Minister strongly maintains. Quite to the contrary, this will make it even more difficult for mothers to combine work and family life and will certainly not enhance female occupational levels. Similarly, if the government discontinues the newly established National Fund, once more the responsibility for long-term care policies will rest only with the regions. Needless to say, this will negatively affect the amount of support that families can receive for their frail elderly members and will worsen equity of access to long-term care services across the country.

A more positive approach emerges from the measures which the Italian government introduced following the outbreak of the international financial crisis at the end of 2008, particularly decree-law no. 185 of 29 November 2008, which Parliament converted into law no. 2 of 28 January 2009. This piece of legislation allocates almost EUR 2 billion for the so-called "family bonus". To place this type of intervention into perspective, one might recall the latest Eurostat data on Member States' distribution of social expenditure by function.[16] According to available evidence, Italy spends only 1.1% of GDP on family allowances compared to an EU 15 weighted average of 2.2%. In short, this policy field is under-funded and the government's decision to intervene in this field appears most appropriate. Further, evidence presented in the 2008 Demography Report by the European Commission shows that in Italy 41% of large families (two-adult households with three or more children) are at-risk-of poverty as compared to 20% of the entire population. Not surprisingly, according to Eurobarometer,[17] Italy displays one of the lowest levels of satisfaction with public support for families with children: in detail, according to survey data, 62% of Italians are not very satisfied or not at all satisfied with public intervention in this policy area. But what exactly does law 2/2009 envisage to support households with children? First of all, intervention is exclusively limited to 2009. According to article 1, the family bonus consists of a lump sum ranging from a minimum of 200 to a maximum of 1,000€ depending on disposable income and size of the family (see Table 10). The measure does not specifically refer to children but to family members dependent on the household head. According to calculations

---

[15] To understand the rationale of these measures, one needs to consider that the Government's stated primary goal is to balance the budget by 2011.

[16] Eurostat (2008), *Social protection in the European Union,* Statistics in focus 46/2008, p. 5.

[17] Eurobarometer no. 247 *Family life and the needs of an ageing population.*

Table 10 Main features of the Italian "family bonus" for 2009, as defined by decree-law
185/2008

Lump sum family bonus	Size of the household	Income threshold
200€	Single person 65 years and over	15,000€
300€	Two-person households	17,000€
450€	Three-person households	17,000€
500€	Four-person households	20,000€
600€	Five-person households	20,000€
1,000€	Households with more than five persons	22,000€

by Baldini and Pellegrino (2009) the bonus will positively affect a considerable
proportion of families in the first five deciles of national income distribution with as
much as 54% of total spending benefiting the Southern part of the country – that is to
say the area in which poverty is more heavily concentrated, especially among large
families.[18]

However, as pointed out in the political and academic debate, the government's
approach suffers from a number of shortcomings. First, procedures to apply for the
benefit are rather complicated and timing is very stringent; but even more important,
instead of extending and improving the existing system of family benefits – which
is far from providing universal coverage – the government opts for adding a further
temporary benefit which is totally unrelated to the existing system.[19]

What is the final message? So far, neither centre-left nor centre-right governments have been able to update the old Fordist model and determine the way out.
Any attempt to seriously re-design the social protection system inevitably entails
challenging existing entitlements, and finding the resources for housing support,
childcare services and family allowances, as well as funding adequate protection
against poverty and unemployment. Given the current distribution of Italian social
expenditure and the practical impossibility of further exacerbating fiscal and contributory pressure, pensions appear the first candidate of any redistributive effort.
However, for the time being this remains academic wishful thinking, at least until the
country and its political leadership start looking ahead instead of looking backwards.
Italy appears to be a country largely dominated by "family politics" but certainly not
by "family policies".

---

[18] Baldini and Pellegrino calculated that almost 40% of Southern families will receive the "family
bonus".

[19] To increase even further the overall fragmentation of family benefits, the government envisaged
the distribution of a pre-paid electronic card to an estimated total number of 300,000 families below
the poverty line, with a child under 3 years of age. The pre-paid electronic card is worth 40€ per
month, starting in October 2008 and expiring in December 2009. At present no renewals are in
sight. The monthly instalments are supposed to be used to pay electricity and gas bills, as well as
food in department stores under contract.

Appendix

Table 11 Monthly family benefits for the worker's children, wife and parents, by occupational sector, 1952, 1956, 1958 (figures in current lira)

	Industry	Tobacco	Handicraft[a]		Trade	Banking[a]		Insurance	Tax collection services on contract[a]		Agriculture[a]	
For each child												
1952	3,978	3,978	1,898	1,950	3,978	884	1,053	2,288	884	1,053	1,170	2,860
1956	4,342	4,342	3,120	3,978	4,342	5,356	5,356	3,120	4,160	4,160	1,560	3,796
1958	4,628	4,342	3,120	3,978	4,628	5,356	5,356	3,900	4,160	4,160	2,340	4,342
For the wife or the disabled husband												
1952	2,600	2,600	1,404	1,456	2,600	884	1,066	2,054	884	1,066	962	1,820
1956	3,016	2,808	2,210	2,600	3,016	5,356	5,356	2,498	2,808	2,808	1,300	2,418
1958	3,302	3,016	2,210	2,600	3,302	5,356	5,356	2,990	2,808	2,808	1,690	3,016
For each parent												
1952	1,430	1,430	1,209	1,248	2,600	832	936	1,716	832	936	780	1,430
1956	1,430	1,430	1,430	1,430	3,016	5,356	5,356	1,716	1,430	1,430	1,040	1,430
1958	1,430	1,430	1,430	1,430	3,302	5,356	5,356	1,716	1,430	1,430	1,300	1,430

[a]The two separate columns refer to blue-collar and white-collar workers, respectively.
Source: Paretti and Cerbella (1958, tav.31 e 32)

References

Baldini, M., & Pellegrino, S. (2009). *Si fa presto a dire Bonus*. Retrieved from http://www.lavoce.info

Battistoni, L. (Ed.). (2005). *I numeri delle donne 2005*. Quaderni Spinn, 17, Rome.

Bernardi, F. (2005). Public policies and low fertility: Rationales for public intervention and a diagnosis for the Spanish case. *Journal of European Social Policy, 15*(2), 123–138.

Bertolini, S. (2006). La conciliazione per le lavoratrici atipiche. *Economia & Lavoro, 15*(1).

Bettio, F., & Plantanega, J. (2004). Comparing care regimes in Europe. *Feminist Economics, 10*(1), 85–113.

Bimbi, F., & Trifiletti, R. (Eds.). (2006). *Madri sole e nuove famiglie. Declinazioni inattese della genitorialità*. Rome: Edizioni Lavoro.

Camera dei deputati. (1957). Relazioni della Commissione Parlmentare d'Inchiesta sulle condizioni dei lavoratori. *Previdenza Sociale*, XI.

Cittadinanzattiva. (2007). *Gli asili nido comunali in Italia, tra caro rette e liste d'attes*. Retrieved from http://cittadinanzattiva.it

European Commission. (2008). *Child poverty and well-being in the EU*. Brussels: European Commission.

Fargion, V. (2004). Tra Scilla e Cariddi. Le politiche sociali dei governi di centro sinistra. *Polis, 3*, 383–412.

Fargion, V. (1997). *Geografia della cittadinanza sociale in Italia*. Bologna: Il Mulino.

Ferrera, M. (1996). The 'southern model' of welfare in social Europe. *Journal of European Social Policy, 6*(1), 17–37.

Ferrera, M. (2008). *Il fattore D*. Milan: Mondatori.

Franco, D. (1993). *L'espansione della spesa pubblica in Italia*. Bologna: Il Mulino.

ISTAT. (2006a). *Natalità e fecondità della popolazione residente: caratteristiche e tendenze recenti*. Rome: ISTAT.

ISTAT. (2006b). *Avere un figlio in Italia*. Rome: ISTAT.

ISTAT. (2007a). *Essere madri in Italia*. Rome: ISTAT. Retrieved from http://www.istat.it

ISTAT. (2007b). *La povertà relativa in Italia nel 2006*. Rome: ISTAT.

Lo Conte, M., & Prati, S. (2003). *Maternità e partecipazione femminile al mercato del lavoro. Un'analisi della situazione professionale delle neo-madri*. Rome: ISTAT.

Lo Conte, M., Prati, S., & Talucci, V. (2003). *Le strategie di conciliazione e le reti formali e informali di sostegno alle famiglie con figli piccolo*. Rome: ISTAT.

Masini, C. A. (1962). Il sistema degli assegni familiari in Italia e l'opportunità di una riforma. *Previdenza Sociale, 18*(1).

Ministero del Lavoro, della Salute delle Politiche Sociali. (2008). *Libro verde sul futuro del modello sociale. La vita buona nella società attiva*, 25. Retrieved from www.lavoro.gov.it

Naldini, M. (2006a). *Le politiche sociali in Europa*. Rome: Carocci.

Naldini, M. (2006b). Trasformazioni lavorative e familiari: soluzioni di policy in diversi regimi di welfare. *Economia e Lavoro, 40*(1), 73–90.

Nunin, R., & Vezzosi, E. (Eds.). (2007). *Donne e famiglie nei sistemi di welfare. Esperienze nazionali e regionali a confront*. Rome: Carocci.

Paretti, O., & Cerbella, A., (1958). *Sintesi della Previdenza Sociale*. Naples: Pironti e Figli Editori.

Saraceno, C. (1998). *Mutamenti della famiglia e politiche sociali in Italia*. Bologna: Il Mulino.

Saraceno, C. (2005). *L'arduo incontro tra donne e lavoro*. Retrieved from http://www.lavoce.info

Saraceno, C., & Brandolini, A. (Eds.). (2008). *Povertà e benessere. Geografia delle disuguaglianze in Italia*. Bologna: Il Mulino.

Saraceno, C., & Leira, A. (Eds.). (2008). *Childhood: changing contexts*. Bingley: Emerald.

Senato della Repubblica. (1961). III Legislatura. *Atti Parlamentari-Resoconti delle Discussioni* (Vol. 25, pp. 21–815). Rome: Senato della Repubblica.

The Erosion of "Familism" in the Spanish Welfare State: Childcare Policy Since 1975

Celia Valiente

Introduction

Social policy in Mediterranean countries, including Spain, is characterized by "familism." Official policy in this region reinforces the historically crucial role of the family as welfare provider. This chapter argues that although "familism" is still a central feature of the Spanish welfare state, a serious erosion of "familism" is taking place. This erosion is evident in increased state and/or market provision of care services, which were traditionally provided by the family, and is illustrated here with an examination of childcare policies in Spain since 1975. Currently preschool attendance rates in Spain are among the highest in the European Union (EU) for children aged three, four, and five (97%, 98%, and 100% respectively in academic year 2006–2007; Ministerio de Educación, Política Social y Deporte, 2008). Because preschool in Spain is primarily all-day, Spanish children aged 3–5 are being cared for by school staff during an important share of the workday. Ever increasing female employment rates are possibly the main factor causing the reduction of "familism." By supporting options that relieve families of some childcare responsibilities, political and social actors are also central to the decline of "familism." These influences on the Spanish welfare state are the focus of this chapter.

This chapter is divided into five sections. In the first section, the analytical framework of this study is presented. Next the selection of the empirical case, childcare policies in Spain after 1975, is justified. In the third section, preschool policies in postauthoritarian Spain are described. The fourth section includes data on the increasing presence of women in the Spanish labor market. Finally, the fifth section

C. Valiente (✉)
Universidad Carlos III, Madrid, Spain
e-mail: valiente@polsoc.uc3m.es

The research contained in this paper is part of a larger international and comparative research project on "Gender and citizenship in multicultural Europe: The impact of the contemporary women's movements (FEMCIT)" financed by the European Commission's Sixth Framework Program (EC contract number 028746-2).

M. Ajzenstadt, J. Gal (eds.), *Children, Gender and Families in Mediterranean Welfare States*, Children's Well-Being: Indicators and Research 2, DOI 10.1007/978-90-481-8842-0_6, © Springer Science+Business Media B.V. 2010

analyzes the role played by political and social actors in the area of childcare policy. Bibliography and published documents and statistics are the main sources of this chapter.

Analytical Framework

According to Esping-Andersen's typology of welfare states in industrial capitalist countries, the Spanish welfare state (and that of other Mediterranean countries) is classified as continental.[1] Social rights, in continental welfare states, are linked to occupational categories and status. For example, different categories of workers are eligible for different insurance schemes. Salaried workers and their dependents are the beneficiaries of the main social programs. Furthermore, redistributive effects of social policies in continental welfare states are minimal. This results in a certain degree of de-commodification, which means, that to some extent, "individuals, or families, can uphold a socially acceptable standard of living" independent of their participation in the market (Esping-Andersen, 1990). The continental welfare state aims at reinforcing the traditionally crucial role of the family as welfare provider. Thus, the state tends to intervene only when the capacity of the family to act as social provider is exhausted and in these cases the provision of welfare benefits is mainly public (Esping-Andersen, 1990).[2]

The Spanish welfare state, like other continental welfare states, is mainly transfer-oriented and offers very few care services (Guillén & Petmesidou, 2008; León, 2007). Historically, political and social actors assumed that care was provided by the family unit. This is one of the factors that contributes to the overwhelmingly "familial" character of the Spanish welfare state (Ferrera, 2007; Moreno, 2008; Moreno Mínguez, 2004; Naldini, 2003; Flaquer, 2004; León, 2002).[3] In most traditional societies, women provide the majority of care for needy populations like the elderly, disabled, ill and small children (Orloff, 1993). Therefore, in societies where the provision of care is by the family unit, women, on an unpaid basis, provide most of the necessary care.

Notwithstanding the above, several changes have been evident in the Spanish welfare state. For example, in the last few decades, private pensions and private

---

[1] Esping-Andersen (1990, pp. 3–4) analyzes the variation across welfare states along three dimensions: the type of social rights; the type of stratification that the welfare state produces; and the interrelation of the state, the market, and the family in the provision of welfare.

[2] Two other types of welfare states exist in the classification made by Esping-Andersen (1990, pp. 7–28): the social democratic and the liberal welfare states. Social democratic welfare states, which exist in Nordic countries, are characterized by wide universal benefits, a high level of de-commodification and social programs that are directed to all social classes. The purpose of social policy in this type of welfare state is to attain equality. The state provides generous care services for children, the elderly, and others in need of care.

[3] Most authors argue that "familism" is a central feature of the Spanish welfare state, regardless of whether authors classify the Spanish state as belonging to the cluster of continental welfare states or to a fourth cluster of Mediterranean welfare states.

health insurance schemes have been developed (Chuliá, 2007; Guillén & Petmesidou, 2008). In addition, historically, "familism" developed because many Spanish housewives were available to take care of their relatives on a full-time basis. While "familism" is still a feature of the Spanish welfare state, this traditional structure is being seriously challenged by increased female participation in the work force (Climent, 2008). This change in the social structure that made "familism" possible directly correlates with a demand for public or publicly funded care services and/or private care schemes provided by the market.

In addition to women's participation in the labor market, other factors may challenge "familism," including the behavior of some political and social actors. Let me focus on the Catholic Church. Spain is a culturally homogeneous Catholic country. After the expulsion of Jews in 1492 and of Muslims soon afterwards, no significant religious community other than the Catholic community has been openly active in Spain. The majority of adult Spaniards consider themselves Catholic (75.8% in July 2008).[4] The number of practicing Catholics is significantly lower than the number of self-declared Catholics: 14.7% of those self-declared Catholics or believers of other religions affirmed that they attended religious services (excluding social events such as weddings, first communions, or funerals) almost every Sunday or public holiday, and 1.9% attended on various days during the week (Centro de Investigaciones Sociológicas, 2008). In Spain specifically, the Catholic Church has played a significant role in the development of the welfare state.

Literature on the origin and development of welfare states in Western countries has privileged the study of socio-economic development and class politics as primary forces causing the establishment and expansion of social policy (Castles, 1994; Daly, 1999; van Kersbergen, 1995). While the role played by organized religion in social policy making has received less attention, the literature identifies Christian democratic parties as principal actors in the translation of Catholic social doctrine into actual social policy making (Morgan, 2006; van Kersbergen, 1995).[5] However, in postauthoritarian Spain, the Church has no direct political representation, because no major Christian democratic party or trade union exists (Casanova, 1993).

Existing literature on this subject argues that the influence of Catholicism on social policy making is complex. At certain points in history a correlation has been found between Catholicism and the level of social security transfer expenditure (Castles, 1994). Catholic social doctrine has three preferences regarding the sort of social policy to be implemented and thus indirectly influences the type of social policy employed in predominantly Catholic countries like Spain. First of all, Catholic social doctrine holds that social provision should be implemented by civil society organizations (especially those of the Catholic Church). Secondly, social provision should preserve status differences in society, for instance, through different schemes

---

[4] In the same opinion poll 2.2% of the interviewed identified themselves as belonging to other religions, 13.1% as nonbelievers, 6.4% as atheist, and 2.4% did not answer.

[5] For a critique of the importance given to Christian democratic parties by this literature, see Castles (1994, pp. 23–24) and Daly (1999, p. 106).

for different types of workers. Lastly, rather than providing care services to families and replacing their role in care provision, social provision should help families care for their members by providing them with income insurance in case the primary wage earner is unable to earn a sufficient income in the labor market. In addition, the Catholic hierarchy has historically supported the view that married women belong in their homes taking care of their relatives, and thus maintains that social policy should not interfere but instead reinforce this traditional role (Castles, 1994; Daly, 1999; Morgan, 2006; van Kersbergen, 1995). Overall, according to the comparative literature on the origins and development of welfare states in postindustrial countries, the Catholic Church has historically supported "familism" by demanding that social policy bolsters the role of women as primary caregivers within their households.

Selection of the Empirical Case

Here the case of childcare is chosen to analyze the level of "familism" in Spanish social policy due to the fact that children need constant (or almost constant) supervision. Between the mid-1930s and 1975, Spain was governed by a right-wing authoritarian regime headed by General Francisco Franco. A transition to democracy followed the dictatorship. Here only postauthoritarian Spain is analyzed because childcare policies established before 1975 were formulated in a different political regime and therefore by different political and social actors than in contemporary democratic Spain.

While some welfare state studies do include education policy (see for instance Castles, 1989; Esping-Andersen, 2007) most research on the welfare state has not considered education policy. However, like other social policies, education may help erode social inequalities. Moreover, in some cases such as Spain, preschool works as a functional, although imperfect, equivalent to childcare services for children of certain ages. Therefore, education should not be ignored in the study of social policy and here education policy will be examined as part of the welfare state.

In addition, the study of childcare and education policy offers an opportunity to study the impact of organized religion on social policy. In contemporary Western countries, states and churches have fought for the control of the education system. Therefore, the study of organized religion is especially important to understanding education policy.

Childcare Policies in Spain After 1975

Childcare can be considered in terms of labor market, gender equality, or education policy. In Spain education has always been the predominant rationale for childcare. Historically, the main services provided for children less than 6 years of age have been all-day preschools. These services were either directly provided by the state or by the market, with state funding. At the central state level, the Ministry of Education regulated these services, with the education department of regional governments later taking control of regulation on the local level. Classes for children under six were frequently located in schools where education for other age levels was offered. Staff members with certified pedagogical credentials were responsible for children aged five and under. Preschool hours and holidays were similar to general school hours and holidays.

Since 1975, the main change in childcare policy has been an increase in the supply of public preschool programs for children not eligible for mandatory schooling (those under 6 years of age). These programs are free of charge, full-day, and administered by education authorities. The absolute number and proportion of children who attend public preschool programs in Spain has increased significantly since 1975. While this type of public preschool was attended by 347,026 children younger than six in the 1975–1976 academic year, by the 2007–2008 academic year this figure had tripled to 1,041,426 children. Seen from another perspective, in the 1975–1976 academic year more than a third (38%) of children enrolled in preschool education attended public centers. In the 2007–2008 academic year this proportion was nearly two-thirds (64%). The expansion of the supply of places in public childcare centers has taken place in a context characterized by the existence of a private sector. In the 1975–1976 academic year the number of children enrolled in private preschool education was 573,310, while in the 2006–2007 academic year the figure was 579,089 (calculated by the author from data contained in: Instituto Nacional de Estadística, 1977; Ministerio de Educación y Ciencia, 2007; provisional data for academic year 2007–2008).

In part as a result of this policy, Spanish preschool attendance rates (including both public and private centers) for 3-, 4-, and 5-year-olds are among the highest in the EU at 97, 98, and 100% respectively (academic year 2006–2007; Ministerio de Educación, Política Social y Deporte, 2008). For instance, in the 2004–2005 academic year the participation rate of 3-year-old children in Spanish pre-primary or primary education (95%) was exceeded only by those of Belgium (100%), France and Italy (97% in both countries), and was 23 points higher than the EU-27 average (72%) (Ministerio de Educación y Ciencia, 2007). Conversely, the proportion of Spanish children age two or younger cared for in public or private centers is comparatively low: 5% for children younger than 1 year, 17% of children aged 1 year, and 33% for those 2 years old (academic year 2006–2007 – Ministerio de Educación, Política Social y Deporte, 2008) (see comparative data in Morgan, 2008, pp. 31–32).

Besides the expansion of the supply of public preschool programs, after the democratization of Spain, territorial decentralization has been another significant change in the area of childcare policy. Under Franco, the state was highly centralized, but during the transition to democracy, a broad process of devolution of powers from the central state to the regions (less so to municipalities) began. Since the early 1980s, some regional governments have acquired responsibilities previously assigned to the central state (for instance, education). The process of decentralization of all authority over education to all regions was completed in 2000.[6]

Spain is unique in its provision of educational services for children under the age eligible for mandatory education. Some countries surrounding Spain have a two-track system; one track consisting of education programs aimed at preparing children for mandatory school and another track consisting of childcare services aimed at helping parents juggle the responsibilities of work and family. These services are not administered and/or regulated by education authorities. This two-track system exists in Germany (Scheiwe, 2009) and the United Kingdom (Penn, 2009). While full-day preschool services are the norm in Spain, they are not the universal norm in Western countries. Half-day preschool services are common in the United Kingdom, Germany, Austria, and Poland (Hagemann, Allemann-Ghionda, & Jarausch, 2006; Penn, 2009).

A point of clarification is necessary here. The definition of preschool programs as schools rather than childcare centers has limited their utility for working parents. Preschool programs provide solid educational services for children aged 3–5 years. Addressing the educational needs of young children from all social classes is a laudable goal, and its achievement should be celebrated. However, preschool programs cannot be used by parents as perfect substitutes for childcare because preschool holidays are considerably longer than work holidays, and preschool hours are shorter than full-time work hours. Policies other than preschool education that help parents manage work and family responsibilities are seriously underdeveloped in Spain (León, 2007).

Women in the Spanish Labor Market

At the end of Franco's regime, the presence of women in the labor market was modest in comparison to other countries. In Spain in 1974 the level of female participation in the labor force, as a percentage of female population between 15 and 64 years of age, was 33%. This figure was 12 points lower than the European Economic Community (EEC) (45%) and 16 points below the Organization for Economic Cooperation and Development (OECD) average (49%). In contrast, in 1974, male participation in the Spanish labor force, as a percentage of the male population between 15 and 64 years of age, was in Spain 91%. This figure was slightly above both the EEC average (88%) and OECD average (88%) (Organization for Economic Cooperation and Development, 1992). In fact, in 1974, the majority of Spanish women of working age did not work for wages, while an overwhelming majority of Spanish men of working age did. Thus, there were a large number of women available to provide care on a full-time and un-paid basis. A weak presence

---

[6]Other childcare policies such as tax exceptions for childcare expenses are less important than the supply of preschool places in public centers. Because of space constraints, only the latter is analyzed in this chapter.

of women in the labor market is congruent with (however, not exclusively) a welfare state characterized by "familism."

In contrast, in contemporary Spain, a slight majority of working age women participate in the labor market. In the last few decades, the Spanish female employment rate has constantly increased, and now stands at 55%. Historically most Spanish women who did participate in the labor force left when they got married or had their first child. This trend seems to have been reversed as currently many women remain in the labor force after marriage or the birth of their first child. For instance, already in 2000, the employment rates of women aged 25–34 and 35–44, the age groups with the highest numbers of preschool age children, exceeded 50%: 57 and 53% respectively (Eurostat data; Instituto Nacional de Estadística, 2008). Comparatively, while part-time work in the EU(–27) makes up 31% of female employment and 18% of total employment, it is still less widespread in Spain: 23 and 12% respectively. This indicates that while the female employment rate in Spain (55%) is still below the EU(–27) average (59%), most Spanish women who work have full-time jobs which provide them with a higher degree of economic independence and less time to care for others than women in other EU member states, where part-time work is much more prevalent (Romans, 2008; fourth quarter of 2007 data). Therefore, in many Spanish households, there is no longer a woman to provide care on a full-time basis. Medium and high rates of women's participation in the labor force are not congruent with a welfare state characterized by "familism" and are one of the primary causes of the erosion of "familism" in the Spanish welfare state.

Political and Social Actors in the Policy Area on Childcare

Social policy is not simply a reflection of specific social and economic circumstances. Social policy is influenced by political and social actors which react to social and economic conditions in different ways. Therefore, the study of the role played by political and social actors is crucial to understand social provision.

As previously noted, Spanish childcare policy has always been mainly an education policy independent of the political regime that governed the country. When Franco died in 1975, the central state already had a limited preschool policy regarding children under the age eligible for mandatory education. The Ministry of Education already functioned as the principal institution to formulate policy in this sphere. Sites and staff, although limited, also already existed to implement this policy in the form of preschool teachers and classes for children under six in public schools. After 1975, central state policy makers, and later regional authorities, found it easier to expand what was already in place than to invent a completely new policy. In fact, following the transition to democracy, the supply of public preschool centers has been expanded by parties with various ideological platforms, each for its own reason, while in office at the central state level. These included the center-right coalition of parties under the Union of the Democratic Center (*Unión de Centro Democrático*, UCD) up to 1982, the social-democratic Spanish Socialist Workers'

Party (*Partido Socialista Obrero Español*, PSOE) between 1982 and 1996, the conservative People's Party (*Partido Popular*, PP) between 1996 and 2004, and again the PSOE since then. In the 1970s and 1980s, public preschool availability was expanded especially for children aged four and five, while in the 1990s and after 2000 places were also increased for children aged three.

Governments formed by the UCD, PSOE, and PP have understood preschool services as a necessary means to economic development through human capital. Most EU(–15) member states are economically more developed than Spain. All three governments held that one of the reasons for Spain's relatively stagnant level of economic development was due to an education deficit. The social-democratic PSOE promoted public preschool mainly to diminish class inequality. Historically, access to nonmandatory education was sharply differentiated by class (de Puelles Benítez, 1999; McNair, 1984; Medina, 1976). Furthermore, in the context of strong electoral competition from the PSOE, the conservative PP did not want to be seen by the electorate as a party that defended the interests of affluent citizens, who tend to use private childcare and preschool programs (Valiente, 2003), and thus maintained and increased the supply of publicly supported preschool. For the same reasons, regional governments of different ideological platforms continued to expand public preschool programs when the authority over education was transferred from central state to regional control.[7]

The Catholic Church is a key player in education in Spain, controlling the majority of private centers. Private centers provide educational services to approximately a third of nonuniversity age students. In general, in postauthoritarian Spain, the Catholic Church has been interested in the expansion of education, provided that a substantial part of it is private and subsidized by the state. In the last three decades, the Church has continuously demanded, and obtained, subsidies for provision of private education, including preschool services. In fact, most private provision of nonuniversity education is subsidized by the state. In the 2004–2005 academic year 84% of nonuniversity students in private education were enrolled in subsidized centers (*centros privados concertados*).[8] In the same academic year, 72% of nonuniversity aged students in subsidized private education attended religious centers. State subsidies are an important source of income for providers of private education. On average, in the 2004–2005 academic year, the state provided 75% of the total expenses of subsidized private centers (Instituto Nacional de Estadística, 2007). Up to the 1990s, the state subsidized mainly private mandatory education, but since then the state has increasingly subsidized private preschool education as well.

---

[7] However, some regional governments were more committed to public preschooling than others. Because of space constraints, regional variations are not analyzed here.

[8] In exchange for state funding, if the number of applicants exceeds the number of places subsidized private centers must use the same criteria as public centers to select students. They must also supply education free of charge (this does not include extracurricular activities, school meals, or school textbooks) and they must allow parents, students, and school staff to participate in school decision-making.

The Catholic Church of Spain pursued state subsidies for its schools and preschools in a specific political context. Contemporary Spain belongs to the group of Western countries with secularized policies and societies. The imperfect separation of Church and state in Spain is reflected in its constitution. According to Article 16, Spain is a nondenominational state based on religious freedom. Nevertheless, this very same Article also states that "public authorities will keep in mind the religious beliefs of Spanish society," that is, Catholicism. Article 16 refers to the advantage gained through the cooperation between the state, the Catholic Church, and the remaining denominations. The special treatment of the Catholic Church by the state is mainly reflected in important state transfers, tax exemptions, and financial support to most Catholic schools, hospitals, centers of social action and patronage for the arts. Thus, the Catholic Church in Spain is not self-supporting but depends on state financing for its economic survival. The Catholic Church accepted the principle of nonconfessionality of the Spanish State and the constitutional regulation of state–church relations (Bedoya, 2006; Casanova, 1993; Linz, 1993).

By successfully obtaining subsidies for private schools and preschools, the Catholic Church satisfied two of the preferences of Catholic social doctrine. First of all, part of state educational policy is administered by confessional private schools, organizations controlled by the Church. Second, access to private education is generally related to social class (with certain exceptions). Thus, the existence of a private education sector means the preservation of status differences within society.[9]

Contrary to the claim in the literature on the origin and development of welfare states, in the last three decades the Catholic hierarchy has not vocally or continuously argued that mothers should take responsibility for the care of their children at home. An explanation for the position of the Catholic Church on this matter is not clearly evident. Three tentative explanatory factors exist. First of all, it is likely that the fact that the Spanish Church controls a significant portion of nonuniversity education made the Church hierarchy more interested in the expansion of this sector, in the form of early childhood education, than in promoting care responsibilities on behalf of mothers of young children. Secondly, in many postindustrial countries the Catholic Church staffed its schools mainly with its own human resources: priests and nuns who were paid below market rates. In many of these countries the number of priests and nuns dramatically decreased in the 1960s and 1970s. This loss of human resources forced the Catholic Church in many countries to alter the educational structure of their schools and find financial resources with which to pay its new secular teachers at market rates (Castles, 1989). It is possible that this turn of events encouraged the interest of the Spanish Catholic Church in state subsidies with which to pay its new staff.

---

[9] In postauthoritarian Spain, the Catholic Church has also consistently pursued other policy objectives on education. For example, the Church has demanded that the state grant religion studies academic status in the school curriculum (Bonal, 2000, pp. 205–206; McNair, 1984, p. 144).

Lastly, it is important to consider the Catholic Church as an international organization with international policy. Since the nineteenth century and during many decades of the twentieth century, with varying degrees of intensity, Papal encyclicals such as *Rerum Novarum* (Leo XIII, 1962 [1891], p. 610), *Casti Connubii* (Pius XI, 1962 [1930], pp. 1625–1626), or *Quadragesimo Anno* (Pius XI, 1962 [1931], pp. 639–640) and other papal documents (Pius XII, 1962 [1945]) defined motherhood not only as the main family duty of women but also as women's main obligation towards society. According to the Catholic Church, the married women's place was in the home. Some of these texts vehemently condemned married women's work outside the home equating it with the destruction of family life and social fabric (Valiente, 1997). However, in the area of gender and sexuality issues, since the Papacy of John Paul II (1978–2005), the priority of the Catholic Church has been the fight against homosexuality and reproductive rights (contraception and abortion). The focus on these priorities moved the Catholic Church away from other issues, such as married women's employment outside the home, against which the Catholic Church had historically mobilized.

In addition women have become increasingly active in organizations of civil society whether as part of women's movements or in mixed associations. Thus, women constitute a visible electorate that politicians often take into consideration when calculating what policies to support or oppose. Women have a large presence in civil society, for example, on average women outnumber men in Third Sector organizations dedicated to social causes (Pérez Díaz & López Novo, 2003).

Two branches of the women's movement have relatively recently gained influence. The first branch is composed of housewives' organizations, widows' associations, mothers' movements, and cultural and religious associations. This branch is currently thriving in terms of number of members and degree of activity (Ortbals, 2004). The second branch which is explicitly feminist (hereafter referred to as the feminist movement) emerged in Spain in the late 1960s and early 1970s in the period of liberalization of the authoritarian political regime. Many of the first feminists were active in the opposition to the dictatorship, where they encountered illegal left-wing political parties and trade unions. These bodies have been the (uneasy) allies of the feminist movement ever since (Threlfall, Cousins, & Valiente, 2005). Many feminists mobilized within both feminist groups of civil society and left-wing political parties. When these groups reached power, feminist activists and leaders occupied decision-making positions in the state and advanced an agenda of gender equality. In addition, feminists within left-wing political parties endlessly pressurized male activists and leaders to take gender equality into consideration when choosing their policy objectives (Threlfall et al., 2005). The feminist movement has also intervened in the gender equality policy area mobilizing public opinion in favor of the need to improve women's status (Trujillo Barbadillo, 1999).

Feminists in western countries including Spain have demanded childcare services. However in Spain, the existence of the right-wing authoritarian regime moved Spanish feminists away from issues such as motherhood and childcare. Since the transition to democracy, childcare has been an issue of medium priority for the feminist movement. After 40 years of being inundated with the idea of mothering and caring as the most important task in women's lives, after the dictatorship Spanish feminists were not interested in focusing on issues of motherhood and child-rearing. Women's liberation was then understood as opening the range of concerns that define women's lives, such as waged work, political participation, and control of their bodies. This definition carefully skirts the place of motherhood and childcare in the life of the newly liberated Spanish women (Valiente, 2003).

Even though childcare has not been a top priority for the feminist movement throughout the postauthoritarian period, preschool is seen by important sectors of public opinion not only as an education policy but also as a policy favorable to women. Because an increasing number of women have joined the workforce and preschool helps parents combine work and family, an expansion of public preschool services is perceived by broad sectors of the citizenry as a policy that helps women. Decreasing public preschool financing is interpreted as a policy against women and rarely viable in Spain where women form an ever increasing part of civil society.

Conclusion

Since 1975 the main childcare public policy in Spain has been an ever increasing supply of full-day, public (or publicly funded) preschool free of charge. Although this policy existed before 1975, it was considerably less developed than it is today. As a result today nearly all Spanish children aged three to five are cared for by school staff during the majority of the workday. This contradicts traditional policy regarding care in "familistic" welfare states; care for those who require it is usually provided by family members. The main cause of the decline of "familism" is most probably the increase in women's participation in the Spanish labor market. Another causal factor is the role played by political and social actors in the area of education. These actors include, among others, the Catholic Church and women's movements.

The role of the Catholic Church is of particular interest because in Spain it is not playing its usual role as defined by comparative literature on the origin and development of welfare states. While historically the Catholic Church supported policy congruent with "familism," for instance, by promoting married women's place in the home, in Spain today the Catholic Church has actually encouraged the increase in childcare options outside the home. Thus, the role of organized religion merits further research as churches pursue new aims.

The decline of "familism" in the Spanish welfare state is not only occurring in the field of childcare but also in fields such as elderly care. Future studies should investigate whether this decline is taking place with the same degree of intensity, and whether this decline is associated with public or publicly funded care provision or with market solutions (for instance, care provided by immigrant workers). Future research should also investigate factors causing the erosion of "familism." Women's employment and the role played by political and social actors in the expansion of social policies are most likely part of these causal factors. Other factors not explored in this chapter may also be at play, such as changing definitions of family obligations, and must be investigated at length.

References

Bedoya, J. G. (2006). Las cuentas del catolicismo español. *El País, 30*, 43.
Bonal, X. (2000). Interest groups and the state in contemporary Spanish education policy. *Journal of Educational Policy, 15*(2), 201–216.
Casanova, J. (1993). Church, state, nation, and civil society in Spain and Poland. In S. A. Arjomand (Ed.), *The political dimensions of religion* (pp. 101–153). Albany (New York): State University of New York Press.
Castles, F. G. (1989). Explaining public education expenditure in OECD nations. *European Journal of Political Research, 17*(4), 431–448.
Castles, F. G. (1994). On religion and public policy: Does Catholicism make a difference? *European Journal of Political Research, 25*(1), 19–40.
Centro de Investigaciones Sociológicas. (2008). *Estudio 2.769*. Retrieved from www.cis.es
Chuliá, E. (2007). Spain: Between majority rule and incrementalism. In E. M. Immergut, K. M. Anderson, & I. Schulze (Eds.), *The handbook of West European pension politics* (pp. 499–554). Oxford: Oxford University Press.
Climent, S. (2008, April 2–3). *Gender and migration and the legal frame of de-familiarization in the Spanish welfare state*. Paper presented at the conference on Gendering Theories of Citizenship: Europeanization and Care, Roskilde, Denmark.
Daly, M. (1999). The functioning family: Catholicism and social policy in Germany and Ireland. *Comparative Social Research, 18*, 105–133.
De Puelles Benítez, M. (1999). *Educación e ideología en la España contemporánea* (4th ed.). Barcelona: Labor.
Esping-Andersen, G. (1990). *The three worlds of welfare capitalism*. Princeton: Princeton University Press.
Esping-Andersen, G. (2007, April 26–27). *Investing in children and their life chances*. Paper presented at the international conference on Welfare State and Competitivity: The European Experience and the Agenda for Latin America, Fundación Carolina, Madrid.
Ferrera, M. (2007). Democratization and social policy in Southern Europe: From expansion to "recalibration". In Y. Bangura (Ed.), *Democracy and social policy* (pp. 90–113). Basingstoke: Palgrave Macmillan.
Flaquer, L. (2004). La articulación entre familia y el Estado de bienestar en los países del Sur de Europa. *Papers: Revista de Sociología, 73*, 27–58.
Guillén, A. M., & Petmesidou, M. (2008). The public-private mix in Southern Europe: What changed in the last decade? In M. Seeleib-Kaiser (Ed.), *Welfare state transformations: Comparative perspectives* (pp. 56–78). Basingstoke: Palgrave Macmillan.
Hagemann, K, Allemann-Ghionda, C., & Jarausch, K. H. (2006). *International and interdisciplinary research project – The German half-day model: A European Sonderweg*. Retrieved from www.time-politics.com.
Instituto Nacional de Estadística. (1977). *Estadística de la enseñanza en España. Curso 1975–76*. Madrid: Instituto Nacional de Estadística.
Instituto Nacional de Estadística. (2007). *Notas de prensa-19 de julio de 2007: Encuesta de Financiación y Gastos de la Enseñanza Privada, curso 2004–2005*. Retrieved from www.ine.es
Instituto Nacional de Estadística. (2008). *Encuesta de la Fuerza de Trabajo de la UE (UE LFS): Datos europeos*. Retrieved from www.ine.es
Leo XIII. (1962 [1891]). Rerum Novarum. In Acción Católica Española (Ed.), *Colección de Encíclicas y documentos pontificios* (Vol. 1, pp. 595–617). Madrid: Publicaciones de la Junta Nacional.

León, M. (2002). Equívocos de la solidaridad: Prácticas familiaristas en la construcción de la política social española. *Revista Internacional de Sociología, 31*, 137–164.

León, M. (2007). Speeding up or holding back? Institutional factors in the development of childcare provision in Spain. *European Societies, 9*(3), 315–337.

Linz, J. J. (1993). Religión y política en España. In R. Díaz-Salazar & S. Giner (Eds.), *Religión y sociedad en España* (pp. 1–50). Madrid: Centro de Investigaciones Sociológicas.

McNair, J. M. (1984). *Education for a changing Spain*. Manchester: Manchester University Press.

Medina, A. (1976). Problemática de la educación preescolar en España. *Revista de Educación, 247*, 111–134.

Ministerio de Educación y Ciencia. (2007). *Datos y cifras, curso escolar 2007/2008*. Retrieved from www.mepsyd.es

Ministerio de Educación, Política Social y Deporte. (2008). *Estadística de las enseñanzas no universitarias: Resultados detallados del curso 2006–2007*. Retrieved from www.mepsyd.es

Moreno, L. (2008). *The Nordic path of Spain's Mediterranean welfare*. Harvard University-Center for European Studies Working Paper 163.

Moreno Mínguez, A. (2004). El familiarismo cultural en los Estados de bienestar del sur de Europa: Transformaciones de las relaciones entre lo público y lo privado. *Sistema: Revista de Ciencias Sociales, 182*, 47–74.

Morgan, K. J. (2006). *Working mothers and the welfare state: Religion and the politics of work-family policies in Western Europe and the United States*. Stanford: Stanford University Press.

Morgan, K. J. (2008, forthcoming). Towards the Europeanization of work-family policies? The Impact of the EU on policies for working parents. In S. Roth (Ed.), *Gender politics in the expanding European Union: Mobilization, inclusion, exclusion* (pp. 37–59). Oxford and New York: Berghahn.

Naldini, M. (2003). *The family in the Mediterranean welfare state*. London: Frank Cass.

OECD. (1992). *Historical statistics*. Paris: Organization for Economic Cooperation and Development.

Orloff, A. S. (1993). Gender and the social rights of citizenship: The comparative analysis of gender and welfare states. *American Sociological Review, 58*(3), 303–328.

Ortbals, C. D. (2004). *Embedded institutions, activisms, and discourses: Untangling the intersections of women's civil society and women's policy agencies in Spain*. Ph.D. dissertation, Indiana University.

Penn, H. (2009, forthcoming). Public and private: The history of early education and care institutions in the UK. In K. Scheiwe & H. Willekens (Eds.), *Childcare and preschool developments in Europe: Institutional perspectives*. Basingstoke: Palgrave Macmillan.

Pérez Díaz, V., & López Novo, J. P. (2003). *El tercer sector social en España*. Madrid: Ministerio de Trabajo y Asuntos Sociales.

Pius XI. (1962 [1930]). Casti Connubii. In Acción Católica Española (Ed.), *Colección de Encíclicas y documentos pontificios* (Vol. 2, pp. 1609–1640). Madrid: Publicaciones de la Junta Nacional.

Pius XI. (1962 [1931]). Quadragesimo Anno. In Acción Católica Española (Ed.), *Colección de Encíclicas y documentos pontificios* (Vol. 1, pp. 624–658). Madrid: Publicaciones de la Junta Nacional.

Pius XII. (1962 [1945]). La mujer en la actualidad. In Acción Católica Española (Ed.), *Colección de Encíclicas y documentos pontificios* (Vol. 2, pp. 1686–1693). Madrid: Publicaciones de la Junta Nacional.

Romans, F. (2008). Labor market trends 4th quarter 2007 data. *Eurostat DATA in focus: Population and social conditions* 16.

Scheiwe, K. (2009, forthcoming). Institutional factors as obstacles to the expansion of early child-
    hood education in the FRG. In K. Scheiwe & H. Willekens (Eds.), *Childcare and preschool
    developments in Europe: Institutional perspectives*. Basingstoke: Palgrave Macmillan.
Threlfall, M., Cousins, C., & Valiente, C. (2005). *Gendering Spanish democracy*. London and New
    York: Routledge.
Trujillo Barbadillo, G. (1999). *El movimiento feminista como actor político en España: El caso de
    la aprobación de la Ley de despenalización del aborto de 1985*. Paper presented at the Annual
    Meeting of the Spanish Association of Political Science, Granada.
Valiente, C. (1997). *Políticas públicas de género en perspectiva comparada: La mujer trabajadora
    en Italia y España (1990–1996)*. Madrid: Universidad Autónoma de Madrid.
Valiente, C. (2003). Central state childcare policies in postauthoritarian Spain: Implications for
    gender and carework arrangements. *Gender & Society, 17*(2), 287–292.
van Kersbergen, K. (1995). *Social capitalism: A study of Christian democracy and the welfare
    state*. London: Routledge.

Children, Families and Women in the Israeli State: 1880s–2008

Mimi Ajzenstadt

Introduction

Traditional welfare state theories focused on male workers and class conflict pay little attention to the relationship between women, children, and families and the welfare state. Criticizing these works, feminist scholars applied a gendered lens to these relations (Fraser, 1994; Gordon, 1990; Sainsbury, 1999). These scholars focused on the interplay between unpaid care work tied to the family/private sphere and paid care work associated with the public sphere of the labor market.

Various studies show that most Western welfare regimes adopted a male-breadwinner female-homemaker model, which is based on the idea that a women's place is in the home caring for the family and is thus, economically dependent on a male earner (O'Connor, Orloff, & Shaver, 1999). This model is characterized by a gender division of labor: men dedicated themselves to market work and women were occupied in unpaid care and domestic work (O'Connor, 1993). Because they were free from domestic responsibility, men had a privileged position in the labor market (Orloff, 1999). In contrast, due to the demands of domestic care, women were less able to take advantage of their labor power (Western, 1999). Scholars have shown how education, welfare, health, and labor policies were shaped by, and at the same time, reinforced the notion of women's domesticity and dependency (Crompton, 2006).

These works classified models of such relations as part of the various welfare state regimes (familial vs. nonfamilial, strong male breadwinner regime types vs. weak breadwinner regime), and underscored the patriarchal ideology that subordinates "care-giving" to "paid work" in a variety of ways (Blau & Abramovitz, 2004; Sainsbury, 1994). The traditional role of women as caretakers for family members, especially children, is a key factor in processes of policy inclusion and exclusion (Abramovitz, 2000; Lewis, 1992; Lewis & Campbell, 2007).

M. Ajzenstadt (✉)
Paul Baerwald School of Social Work & Social Welfare, The Institute of Criminology,
Faculty of Law, Hebrew University of Jerusalem, 91905 Jerusalem, Israel
e-mail: mimi@mscc.huji.ac.il

M. Ajzenstadt, J. Gal (eds.), *Children, Gender and Families in Mediterranean Welfare States*, Children's Well-Being: Indicators and Research 2, DOI 10.1007/978-90-481-8842-0_7, © Springer Science+Business Media B.V. 2010

Recently, scholars have called for the examination of the mechanisms of inclusion and exclusion of women, families, and children within structural and cultural contexts, linking them to wider social and political debates and processes (Voet, 1998; Yuval-Davis, 1993). As part and parcel of this investigation, they encourage the examination of the public and political discourse surrounding the development and implementation of social polices in order to understand cultural schemes which inform social policy (Lewis & Giullari, 2005). This wider context structures and shapes both policies and perceptions about entitlements of members of various groups in specific societies and the allocation of resources to these groups (Williams, 1995; Gillies, 2005). In this literature, women and children's needs, identities and capacities for fulfilling their assigned roles, are framed according to the society's vision regarding these groups' social role within a specific national context.

This chapter follows these ideas through a historical comparative perspective which sheds light on the ways in which women, children, and families were perceived, and socially and culturally constructed, in Israel (and pre-state Mandatory Palestine or Ottoman Palestine) from the end of the nineteenth century until today. These conceptualizations are contextualized within the wider social-political framework of Israeli society in four different periods, during which debates about the inclusion and exclusion of women, children, and families took place. The chapter highlights the dominant conceptualization, specifying the trajectory of the national context of each of the specified periods.[1]

The Pre-State Period: 1880–1948

Beginning at the end of the nineteenth century, waves of Jewish immigrants came to Palestine, aiming to build a modern Jewish state. The first waves of immigrants resided mainly in small villages working in agriculture. Zionist leaders envisioned women in the ideal family as central to financial earnings and the creation of a healthy moral foundation for all family members. Both contributions were regarded as essential to Zionist aspirations. Women combining work in the field with caretaking responsibilities in the home were seen as a "blessed source for the community as well as for the women themselves" (Stoler-Liss, 2003). In reality, however, women were mainly occupied in traditional female tasks including cooking, doing house work and caring for family members.

During the next 60 years, the Jewish community continued to grow as new waves of immigrants came to Palestine. In this pre-state period, the position of women did not change. While some of them joined the labor force, they were marginalized in their social position as workers and their earnings were minimal (Bernstein,

---

[1] The Arab minority population comprises approximately 20% of the Israeli population. The relations between Arab women, children, and families and the state of Israel are central for scholars of the welfare state. However, it is beyond the scope of this chapter which concentrates only on the Jewish population.

1992). While women's contribution to the work force was not valued, their duty as caregivers and mothers was appreciated and portrayed as a key mission of the development of a Jewish state. The gendered supreme role of giving birth and raising healthy and strong children was embedded in the Zionist ethos which saw settlement in Palestine as a cure to the ills of previous generations. According to Zionist ideology, the prototype religious, European Jew had been impaired in the Diaspora. Centuries of living a traditional Jewish life in dark, crowded, and airless ghettos had affected the health and sexual stamina of the European Jew, making him sick and weak (see discussion in Ajzenstadt & Cavaglion, 2002).

Zionism was seen as a medicine to cure "the degenerative Diaspora's slovenly body, transforming it into a muscular one" (Nordau, 1955, pp. 117–118). Herzl, in his utopian *Altneuland* ([ca. 1902] 1960), envisioned a new nation of healthy, free, serious, and secure Jews upstanding among their brethren and "perfect in their bodies" (pp. 76–85). The pioneers saw the developing of the "new Jew" and thus the new nation as a way of transforming the Jewish community into a sane and strong community. In the 1940s the ethos of the ideal Zionist hero expanded from the image of the pioneer farmer to include the soldier, fighting against those who attempted to undermine the establishment of the new state: "The pioneers are facing huge obstacles: untilled land, deathly swamps, Arabs, hostile authorities (the British mandate) ... [T]hey overcome these hardships holding in the one hand the pure weapon and in the other the plough" (Firer, 1984, p. 15). This image of the new, healthy Jew who fought to defend his community and did not give in to external pressures was constructed as the new hero of Jewish settlement in Palestine. Within this context, mothers were defined as the creators of the new, brave, and healthy Jew (see discussion in Stoler-Liss, 2003). Their role as the biological producers of the nation was established as the inclusive mechanism in the emerging society (see for example Elboim-Dror, 1994).

The significance of motherhood was embedded in the various campaigns of the women's movements established during this time, which demanded the enhancement of woman's status within the Jewish community. Their demands, which were encapsulated in their wider visions of citizenship, cultural positioning and belonging, saw motherhood as a central element in the process of nation building (Katznelson-Rubatchov, 1947). For them, woman's inclusion within society was related to her role as head of the family unit. The creation of a modern Jewish family led by women was seen as an integral part of the creation of the new Jewish state which needed healthy males, healthy children, and healthy families. Adopting a maternal ideology, they saw themselves as playing a central and natural role in a nation fighting for the independence of the Jewish nation (Azaryahu, [1948] 1977). In 1944, Henrietta Szold, who chaired the Social Welfare Department of the Vaad Leumi (General Jewish Council), claimed that the family institution should play a central role in society: "The War will be won on the battlefield ... The Peace must be won in the home, the factory and farm!" (Does it matter? The Hadassa Archive AG 17/pamphlets/Box 1/Child welfare).

This path of inclusion for membership in society was not equal for all women. The majority of the people residing in the small Jewish community in Palestine during the pre-state period were native born or immigrated from Europe or North America (Gelber, 1987). The rest immigrated from North Africa and Asia and were negatively stigmatized by members of the dominant group and were portrayed as primitive, barbaric, sick, unclean, ignorant, and uneducated (Ajzenstadt, 2001; Lissak, 1995). In a pamphlet published by the Hadassah organization towards the end of the 1930s, new immigrants were described as "... these women from the East, from time immemorial ... most of them are very poor and ignorant of personal and social hygiene" (Hadassah, "Out of the Cradle endlessly rocking," The Hadassa Archive RG 17 Ia, Child Welfare Fund). Since this population was viewed as not ready to enter modern society, they were seen as an obstacle to the smooth development to a modern, healthy society. Mothers from this group were not seen as fit to create the familial foundation necessary for the new society. For example, a social worker at that time claimed that those from the Orient could not understand the values of the Western culture because they had not developed sufficiently and thus were not yet ready to productively join the collective (Tahon, 1937).

A host of educational and legal programs targeting these women were developed which aimed to help them internalize the "correct" values and norms appropriate to the emerging society in order to prepare them to become "fit" to be included in society. Members of women's organizations took it upon themselves to teach these women about the rules of sanitation, food preparation, raising children and allowance money in an effort to help the women mature and thus become part of Israeli society in the future (Hirsch, 2008). As part of this project, women activists attempted to instruct new immigrants on how to run the ideal home, which followed modern western cultural norms, and learn how "to build a family where she would be able to fulfill her obligations for the benefit of her husband and children and entire society" (A letter to Sarah Azayahu 1.4.1935, Zionist Archives, 6/2/15).

Uneducated, wayward, and hungry children from poor families were considered as traumatic to society, since: "any function of nation-building should begin with the boys and girls of a land who must be taught early to prepare themselves for a creative adult life" (The Hadassa Archive RG 17 1A). During the Second World War, the mission awaiting Jewish children was expanded to include a national as well as an international mission: "We need to prepare these boys and girls to be fit protectors of the rights of men for which all allied nations are fighting today, and fit co-citizens of that democratic world which we are building for ourselves and generations yet unborn ...they have to be well-fed, well educated and well taken care of" (Does it matter? The Hadassa Archive AG 17/pamphlets/Box 1/Child welfare).

A direct link was drawn between the education of the children and the future of the entire nation. In fact, children were seen as required to undertake the burden of the Zionist revolution and the protection of the family and its normative functioning. This strong relationship between children and the developing community was translated into various programs aimed at enabling women and children to fulfill their expected role and mission. Social workers visited new immigrant mothers and taught them how to take care of their children in order to ensure that they would grow up as healthy individuals ready to serve the nation and the world. The wellbeing of children and the creation of healthy families were aims closely tied to the Zionist project (see for example discussion in Shilo, 2007). Within this context, women's citizenship was further structured by their contribution to this valued national aim.

1950s–1960s: Legal and Social Protection of Mothers

Zionist ideology regarding mothers' roles and their inclusionary paths to society were institutionalized after the State of Israel was established in 1948. Mothers continued to be considered the biological reproducers of the nation and were incorporated into society via this role. According to this citizenship model mothers were socially and culturally defined as reproducing agents of the healthy and moral new generation (Berkovitch, 1997). Their role was marked by the fulfillment of the role of motherhood and thus, domesticity was considered a woman's proper destiny (Rapoport & El-Or, 1997). This image was publicly announced in the explanations by the Minister of Justice of the 1951 Equal Rights Law which aimed to grant equal rights to women. While addressing the Knesset (the Israeli Parliament), he projected the image of the mother as a national producer, emphasizing her divine role:

> During the past generations, the Hebrew Jewish woman was a loyal help mate to the pioneers in our land. She helped in the field and the battle but her main contribution is in the fulfillment of her right and duty to nurture the young generation and educate it to be proud, brave and ready to make sacrifices for the nation. She has an honorable place in our recent history (Israeli Parliament records, Vol. 9, 2004).

Similarly, the first Prime Minister, David Ben-Gurion, conceptualized motherhood as a public role of national significance and described the mother, during the deliberation regarding the same law, as the transmitter of beauty and purity to her sons (see Lahav, 1993).

This esteem afforded mothers was supported by an official state structure aimed at enabling mothers to assume their motherly role while simultaneously participating in the workforce. While the number of women who worked outside the home in the 1950s and 1960s was relatively small (in 1960, 27.3% of the women in the civilian working-age population worked), soon after its independence, Israel enacted the 1954 *Employment of Women Law*. Compared to other labor laws, this law is particularly liberal and advanced (Izraeli, 1992; Raday, 1994). It provides for maternity leave and allows for paid leave during pregnancy and pregnancy-related medical examinations.

The ideology which valued women according to their ability to care for the health and morality of their children was further institutionalized by a law ensuring that state institutions would assume the responsibility for social provisions necessary to enable mothers to fulfill their role. The first article of major social security legislation adopted by Israel in 1953 provided hospitalization and maternity grants. The adoption of this benefit program was justified because of its intent to ensure the health and well-being of mothers and their babies. Furthermore, it aimed to consolidate and support the reproductive role of Jewish women, increase their fertility rate, and reduce mortality levels among Jewish mothers. This national mission was initiated within the context of national concern about the low fertility rate of Jewish women as compared to those of Arab women and the consequential demographic gap between Jews and Arabs (see discussion in Ajzenstadt & Gal, 2001).

The 1970s: Mothers, Work and Children

Following the Six-Day War in 1967, rapid economic growth took place in Israel which led to a sharp increase in consumption. As a result severe labor shortages prevailed. In order to assist the state to meet the demands for workers, the government called upon women to join the labor market (Izraeli, 1992). An analysis of the rhetoric used in the requests for women to participate in the working force shows that they were represented as qualitative human capital who could contribute to the needs of the expanding labor market. This perception was voiced by the Minister of Labor, Yosef Almogi, who regarded women as a valued qualitative group of workers and noted: "The labor power of women has a qualitative significance ... the developed industry needs to adopt technological advances and here the women play an important qualitative role even more than the male workers" (Almogi, 1969, p. 314). The Interministerial Committee for the Encouragement of Female Labor established in 1966, feared that women who internalized the traditional social expectations from them, would be reluctant to leave their primary familial role as care givers and join the labor force. Thus, the committee set out to "examine and recommend sufficient ways and means to encourage women to join the labor market" (The Committee for the Encouragement of Female Labor, 1966, p. 134).

Kohavi (1964), the Director of the Employment and Absorption Section in the Labor Ministry, regarded women as rational human beings who already "provided an important service to the nation as mothers and wives. Now the question is how to attract them to the economy awaiting them," (105). The participation of women in the workforce was elevated during this period to become a national mission and policy makers called on women to join the labor market in order to assist the economy, in need of their experienced hands (Bernstein, 1981).

It may seem that the role of women in Israeli society was elevated by this new economic need and as a result of the perception of women as productive workers. Minister Almogi represented this approach by saying: "women's labor carries with it a social aspect beyond the economic ones. I think that an advanced society can no longer confine woman to her kitchen, advancement and the habit of women to stay at home are not correlated. It is matter of a pride, and of human dignity" (Almogi, 1969, p. 313). Thus, it was acknowledged that women's contribution to society should not be restricted only to the private sphere of the family, but that they could play a central role in the public sphere, where in fact they were needed. This inclusion had the potential to change the paths of women and incorporate them into society, not only via their familial status, but also by their valued participation in the workforce. At first sight it would seem that this approach, which regarded

women as potential workers and contributors to the national wealth and wellbeing, marked a change in the perceptions about women's role on behalf of Israeli
society.

A detailed examination of the policies and the calls to increase women's participation in the labor market reveals, however, that such change in perceptions about
the gendered citizenship model did not take place at that time. Women were seen
only as temporary "helpers" in an emergency situation. The traditional commitment
to raise children and care of family members continued to be considered as the primary role of women. In its various deliberations, the Interministerial Committee
for the Encouragement of Female Labor emphasized that entering the work force
should not replace the main social role of women in a significant way, nor should it
affect child birth in the developing country. Aharon Goldstein from the right-wing
Gahal party requested that everything possible be done so that the child birth rate in
the Israeli family is not reduced (Knesset protocols, 18.2.1970, p. 869). The representative of Agudat Israel, the religious party, was concerned that working women
would stop bearing children, in an expression of preference of work over childrea-
ring and suggested that "every woman who joins the workforce would take it upon
herself to give birth to at least two more children," (Knesset protocols, 18.2.1970,
p. 872).

The Labor Minister promised that the fertility rate of the Jewish nation would not
be harmed by women entering the work force: "We conducted two studies which
show that there is no contradiction between working mothers and the fertility rate,
it will remain the same" (Knesset protocol, 18.2.1970, p. 872). He claimed that it is
the duty of the state to ensure that fertility rates would not be affected: "I admit that
women labor is problematic. First of all we immensely want to increase the birth
rate and thus we do not want to do anything which will interfere with it," (Almogi,
1969, p. 314).

The various speakers in the parliament called on women to extend their national
role and mission and help in both areas. They specified that the state should help
working women care for their children and that domestic responsibilities such as
education of children, caring for husbands, and developing healthy and moral homes
should remain mainly in the hands of the mother. In order to facilitate this the
Minister of Labor proposed to open daycare centers near the workplace, create
flexible working hours and assist in payment of housekeepers for working women
(Almogi, 1969, p. 315).

The state thus encouraged a complex combination of motherhood and worker
roles within a context of shifting some responsibilities of child rearing from the
mother to the state. Indeed, a new infrastructure of daycare centers was developed
to care for the children of working mothers (Bar & Markus, 1977; Sheffer, 1999).
In addition, working mothers were eligible for an approximate 30% subsidy of daycare fees (see Ajzenstadt & Gal, 2001). In this way, women's participation in the
labor market continued to be seen as subordinate to their primary role as mothers
and caregivers. Bearing children and educating them was seen as the ideal role for
women. Motherhood was still considered to be the appropriate path for women's
inclusion within society.

Children and the State

After the establishment of the state of Israel in 1948, waves of immigrants arrived, leading to major demographic and social changes in the population. The Jewish residents, who numbered 650,000, absorbed 740,000 new immigrants between 1948 and 1954 (Lissak, 1999). In 1947, 89.6% of the population was of European origin, compared with only 10.4% from North Africa and Southern Asia. These proportions changed dramatically with the influx of immigrants, the majority coming from Asia and North Africa. Thus, during the 1950s and the 1960s, Israeli social structure comprised of a dominant group, which consisted mainly of Ashkenazi veteran Jews of European descent, as well as Orientals, most of them new immigrants, who were unorganized and were given inferior education and housing (Swirski, 1981).

The strong connection between ethnicity and social class, which was created during the pre-state period, was intensified after the state of Israel was established (Smooha, 1993). During this period, Oriental Jews were alienated and geographically, politically, and socially segregated (see Ajzenstadt, 2002). Their access to education was limited and they usually held low wage, blue collar jobs (Ben-Porath, 1986; Steinberg, 1988).

During the 1970s, various social groups among the Orientals protested against their social, cultural, and economic marginalization (see Bernstein, 1984). These protests led to the rediscovery by the government of the poverty, neglect, and marginalization among a wide range of social groups; most of them Orientals (see discussion in Doron, 1985). The Horovitz committee which was established in 1971 and the Katz committee established in 1973 to investigate issues of poverty reaffirmed these claims, pointing to severe financial neglect and deprivation, mainly among Oriental families (see the discussion in Salzberger, 1995). It was feared that poverty, illiteracy, neglect, and feelings of alienation, experienced by these families and especially their children, would threaten the stability of Israeli society.

Politicians and experts responding to the findings insisted that it was the responsibility of the government to assist children in distress and their families, so they could become productive members of society. The head of the opposition, Menachem Begin, linked the status of children and the project of nation building: "We always were proud of the Israeli youth, who are sun tanned . . . healthy in body and mind . . . Israel owes a better life to the children who were always considered the future generation who should build the nation" (Knesset protocols, 11.7.1973, pp. 3857–3858). Hungry, distressed, and uneducated children would not be able to carry out their role in society and thus, the government took it upon itself to care for them, in order to secure the nation's future. During the second half of the 1970s, a set of social security measures were established, among them universal children allowances were introduced. Moreover, during this time a law providing free high school education was enacted. These initiatives were accompanied with a narrative which clarified the relations between families, children, and the state. The government saw the creation of a nourishing environment for children, which ensured their wellbeing and education, as a national project and mission.

The Mid-1990s: Immigrants, Motherhood, the Family and Welfare

With the enactment of the Single Mother Act in 1992 women's role in society and the relations between mothers and the state in regards to caring for children reemerged on the public stage. The act provided higher social assistance benefits to single mothers, abolished the need for a work test for those with children under the age of seven, and provided them with grants to cover school payments in addition to other benefits (Hacker, 2001). The act was created in the context of the influx of a million immigrants who came to Israel during the 1990s from the former Soviet Union. Of them 13% were families with single mothers and this led to a sharp increase in the number of families with single mothers in Israel (Gordon & Eliav, 1992).

The deliberations about the law were embedded once again within the ethos of the national mission of state building and immigrant absorption. Knesset Member Ora Namir who sponsored the act claimed that society should support mothers who stay at home with their children as it should "grant them the opportunity to raise and educate children to be good, happy and healthy citizens" (Parliament protocols 10.12.1991, p. 1205). She emphasized the state's obligation to create the appropriate conditions for new immigrant mothers arriving in Israel alone with their children. She saw the state as responsible for allowing these women to fulfill their role as mothers and give their children the best available education.

Single mothers were even conceptualized as heroines, as bearing the burdens of child-bearing and rearing despite adverse conditions, and were recognized as contributing to the success of the nation. Knesset Member Nava Arad compared the new immigrants to war widows and to women who were widowed due to terrorist attacks. In the latter cases the state took it upon itself to assist in raising their children and thus, she claimed, should do the same for single mothers. She claimed that in the wake of the wave of new immigrants, Israel should extend a supporting hand to help them and to enable them to exercise their freedom. In this way, motherhood was again cherished and valued and was included in wider national aims.

2002–2003: Families, Women and Children in the Neo-Liberal Regime

During the 1980s a stabilization program which aimed to fight economic instability was adopted. This program marks the beginning of the dominance of neo-liberal ideology in Israel. Neo-liberal economic and social policies were adopted in full by the Sharon government during the first years of the twenty-first century and have been pursued in varying degrees by Israeli governments since then. During this period, a materialistic, individualistic socioeconomic regime, which reduced state intervention, liberalized the capital market and aimed at downsizing the state and minimizing its role in the market, was established (Filc, 2005; Shafir & Peled, 2002).

Moreover, health, education, and welfare services were privatized (Ajzenstadt & Rosenhek, 2000; Razin & Sadka, 1993). At the same time, support for the welfare state was gradually reduced and collective rights were devalued. Furthermore collective bargaining agreements were replaced by individual and special labor contracts.

The adoption of a neo-liberal agenda intensified during the first years of the twenty-first century as a response to the economic recession at that time. This recession was caused by the renewal of violent conflict with the Palestinians (the second Intifada) which led to a reduction in investment in Israel, tourism, and personal consumption (Doron, 2005). In addition, Israel was affected by the downturn of the international economy. Together, these factors led to a rise of unemployment to a rate of more then 10%. Netanyahu, the then Finance Minster, who enjoyed strong support from the then Prime Minister Ariel Sharon, declared a recovery program for the economy which included tax cuts, the reduction of the government's involvement in the economy, and increased privatization of state-owned companies (Filc, 2005; Nitzan & Bichler, 2002). The program consisted of wage reductions and massive layoffs, especially in the public sector workforce (Razin & Sadka, 1993). The government reduced the role of the public sector as an employer, replacing it with the private sector, mainly through an increasing number of temporary-employment agencies (Raday, 1999). Until the 1980s, the Histadrut, the Israel Federation of Labor, was a strong trade union, representing 80% of Israeli employees (Raday, 1999). It played a central role in collective bargaining over employees' wage payment and was highly involved in protecting workers' rights. Starting in the 1980s, however, its social and political strength and its ability to secure workers' rights significantly declined (see for example, Gal & Achdut, 2007).

The economic recovery plan also included cuts in the state budget and the curtailing of various benefit and transfer payments, especially child benefits, unemployment compensation, and income support. In addition, the state adopted stricter eligibility guidelines (Rosenhek, 2004). Finally, Israel joined other countries in tying benefits to increased participation in the labor market. The main initiative was the adoption of welfare-to-work programs. New policies targeted welfare recipients of income support, and thus most of them centered on women who comprised the majority of welfare state clients.

The economic plan had dire consequences for single mothers from the lower strata of society. According to the 1992 Single Parent Act, single mothers were eligible for income support if their children were under the age of seven. According to the new plan, however, only mothers of children under the age of two were eligible for this welfare benefit (Achdut, 2007). In 2002, there were 98,300 single parent families with children up to the age of 17. The mother was the sole parent in 91% of these families (89,200) (Swirski, Kraus, Konor-Atias, & Herbst, 2002). After the introduction of the economic plan, 3,000 single mothers who once had been eligible for benefits were no longer eligible (Shachak, 2003). An additional 45,400 single parent families suffered from an average reduction of 30–33% in their welfare benefits (The National Insurance Institute of Israel, 2002). In addition, the National Insurance Institute of Israel lowered the ceiling of alimony provided for child support in circumstances in which a child's father is unable or unwilling to pay (Warzberger, 2003). Finally, the cancellation of this benefit led to the termination of other payments tied to it, such as public transportation subsidies, professional medical care assistance, and housing rental assistance.

As part of the attempts to reduce welfare spending, the government called upon the unemployed, among them women in general and single mothers in particular to "get out and go to work," framing female participation in the labor market as a means to achieve gender and class equality. Furthermore, it framed female involvement in the workforce as a way to become a productive member of society, deserving of a reasonable standard of life (Ministry of Finance http://www.mof.gov.il/hon/2001/pension/memos/plan2003_pres2.pdf).

Israeli women were required to look for work in order to increase their household income. During the last decade, women's participation in the civil labor market has grown from 27.3% of women of the civilian working-age population participating in 1960 to 51% participation in 2007 (Central Bureau of Statistics, 2008; see also Steir, Lewin-Epstein, & Braun, 2001, pp. 1731–1732). Female workers in Israel are concentrated in traditionally female, secondary sectors of employment. For example, they are employed in food and hospitality services, as well as in the fields of nursing and teaching. The increase in the participation of women in the Israeli work force did not change the existing pattern of occupational gender segregation. In 2005, 54% of women participating in the labor market were employed in traditionally female jobs (The Ministry of Industry, Trade and Labor, 2006). In addition, a gendered wage gap exists in Israel. For example, in 2006 the average gross salary of a female worker was 67% of that of the average salary of a male worker (see Yaish & Kraus, 2003).

These gaps cannot be explained by gender differences in education. In 2005, 77.8% of female workers completed more than 16 years of studies compared to 76.8% of the working males (Halperin-Kaddari & Karo, 2007). Many women work part-time instead of full-time jobs. In 2007, 37% of women as compared to 13% of men were employed in part-time occupations (of less then 35 weekly hours) (http://www.cbs.gov.il/reader/newhodaot/hodaa_template.html?hodaa=20081103). Furthermore, part-time workers are commonly perceived as uncommitted workers and thus, very few hold prime labor market positions (Steir & Lewin-Epstein, 2000). This employment pattern reinforces the marginality of women in the Israeli labor market (Steir, 1998).

Moreover, until the mid-1990s, 60% of the public sector workforce in Israel was female (Raday, 1999). While these women were employed in low-paid clerical and service jobs, they enjoyed job security, decent working conditions, and protected rights (Okun, Oliver, & Khait-Marelly, 2007; Steir & Yaish, 2008). With the decline of employment in the public sector, many women became temporarily employed by employment agencies (Nakar, 2006). Approximately one-third of the workers in government ministries are employed by subcontractors, and 65% of all workers employed through temporary employment agencies or subcontractors are women (Warzberger, 2002). These agencies usually offer low-paid jobs which do not require professional skills and entail limited options for professional mobility.

Women employed through temporary employment agencies do not enjoy the benefits provided to women employed in the public service. These benefits include paid leave for medical care during pregnancy or for the purpose of fertility treatment, or paid leave for the care of a sick child. In addition, women working for temporary employment agencies are not provided with job security during maternity leave and do not enjoy labor union protection (Dagan-Bozaglo, 2007). As union power has weakened, workers in various professions, especially those employed by the private sector, have been left unprotected. Collective bargaining and stable hierarchical structures of promotion have been replaced by individualized pay and a merit system, leaving workers belonging to marginalized groups less protected and with fewer tools for negotiating their pay and other work conditions (Elbashan, 2004). Women employed in temporary employment agencies do not enjoy the privilege of union-negotiated wage contracts and are less likely to know their rights regarding, among others, annual holidays and sick leave, and in general their rights are systematically abused (Becker, Abhasera, & Ziv, 2006). Indeed, recent studies indicate that the rights of many women workers, in general, and mothers in particular in Israel are abused and the impact of labor laws on their work condition is minimal. Fifty-three percent of women who returned to their jobs after maternity leave were moved to another job by the employer. Empirical data points to a steady rise in employers' requests to approve dismissal during pregnancy. Between 2000 and 2005 the number of such requests increased by 33.1% (Tamir, 2007). To convince the Ministry of Industry, Trade, and Employment (the government Ministry responsible for enforcing labor laws) that the discharge is not related to pregnancy, employers cite various excuses including a declining need of manpower in the workplace (in 2002, 26% of the approved requests were granted for this reason), noncompliance on behalf of the employee with workplace rules, or interpersonal problems preventing the employee from cooperating with colleagues, employers, or customers (in 2002, 17% of the approved requests were granted for this latter reason). This practice is underreported, and therefore more alarming, given that employers often choose not to apply to the Ministry and instead openly violate the law by dismissing pregnant women. When discharged, women could appeal to the justice system, but they hardly ever do. The women in these cases are permitted to present their case to the ministry during the process and are allowed to be represented by a lawyer. Few women take advantage of this provision because most are unaware of their rights. Those who are aware of these rights are often unable to finance the necessary legal expenses.

Women's organizations, as well as law school clinics and hotlines advising on welfare- and work-related rights, report a steady increase of women complaining that their rights in the labor market are not secure. In addition to termination of employment during pregnancy, women complain that employers refuse to employ pregnant women or mothers, upon return, effectively forcing them to lose their seniority after maternity leave (Tamir, 2007; Tagar, 2006).

These violations are largely ignored by the Ministry of Industry, Trade, and Employment. The limited access to justice and the marginalized social and economic position of many female workers creates a fertile ground for employers wishing to cut costs and enables them to easily violate labor and employment laws (Davidov, 2007). In addition, according to the Women's Lobby in Israel 19% of women employed through temporary employment agencies were victims of sexual harassment. This figure is higher than the 13% of self-employed women or women employed in public services who were victims of sexual harassment (Tamir, 2007).

The government's demand that women increase their participation in the labor market was not accompanied by protection of their rights or assistance with raising children. Labor market conditions left women to fend for themselves in the free market system, which created obstacles for their successful integration into the workforce. Women were forced to compete over scarce jobs on terms dictated by the market, without the protection that the welfare state traditionally provides against negative market effects.

The economic program in the early twenty-first century was accompanied by heated campaigns which projected the unemployed as symbolic of the ills and failures of past generations and as the epitome of an old tradition of the welfare state rationale, which encouraged dependency on state institutions and thus must be erased. In this context, the welfare system was represented as encouraging and sustaining the laziness of welfare recipients, especially women and single mothers (see Ajzenstadt, 2009). They were described by the government as symptomatic of the evil spirit of the past come back to haunt modern, advanced society and its hard-pressed, tax-paying, deserving citizens. Stelzer (*Ha'aretz*, 17.7.2003, p. A2) represented this argument: "Which kind of society do we want to have here: one in which a growing segment of its population live off welfare, do not work and rely on those who do work hard and groan under the tax burden, or a society whose members are productive, working people who can rely on themselves and do not need favors from anyone?"

Thus the neo-liberal economic plan was defined as part of the modern age, characterized by the spirit of rationalism and subjectivism, and grounded in such values as autonomy and freedom from state intervention. An article posted on Finance Minister Netanyahu's website negates state intervention: "Our society has progressed and changed and most people do not wish to finance any more, this type of single motherhood. ...our society is ready to allocate rights but will not be engaged in intervention and encouragement of those groups" (Bertz http://www.netanyahu.org/xruecu.html).

Public discourse represented welfare recipients as dependent on the state and as incapable. Various Nongovernmental Organizations (NGO), which opposed the economic program, submitted an appeal to the High Court of Justice (BAGATZ 366/03). In 2003, the State Attorney's office responded to this appeal by stating: "a utilitarian analysis of income support and other benefits tied to it, and a comparison to the alternative option of integration in the workforce, leads a rational individual who wishes to maximize his disposable income to choose to remain within the benefit system and avoid joining the labor market (p. 14)." Judge Rivlin responded by encouraging the state to look for alternative measures to remedy the economy instead of choosing the easier path that results in abusing the basic rights of the marginalized. He argued that it is the state's responsibility to examine other options, which are compatible with the vision of "our ancestors who aimed to build a society based on solidarity, caring, and equality" (BAGATZ 366/03, p. 52).

Judge Rivlin's calls were not answered and welfare recipients were not only described as choosing an egoistic option, but they were stigmatized, criminalized, and blamed for abusing the system. The unemployed were portrayed as "chronic," "sick," "defeated" people who were captured in a "poverty trap" from which they could not escape. Government representatives believed that the most efficient way to free those who were caught in this net was to shrink the net, forcing the entrapped to join the labor market which offered limited work opportunities. When these measures led to public protest, Prime Minister Sharon responded, at his address during the 2003 Caesarea conference: "We need to make a deep change in the labor force, we need to touch the most sacred cows, some of which no one has dared to touch since the establishment of the state. As someone who understands something about raising animals, I understand something about cows, and I say it loud and clear: and I am not deterred by their mooing" (3/7/03, p. 2).

Compared to the discourse launched during the 1970s, current policy and the discourse relating to female labor was no longer a discourse emphasizing women's valued contribution to the nation. The discourse was fueled with criminalization and a policy of control and coercion. Single mothers for example, were monitored by a special division of the National Insurance Institute who looked for signs that they clandestinely live with a partner (http://www.yedid.org.il/press.he.asp?id=250). Even the mere suspicion of this kind of relationship led to the abolishment, without warning or notification, of the single mother benefit.

Most importantly, the new economic regime undercut the significance of national symbols which were recently regarded as critical to the well-being and the smooth functioning of the entire social order and the nation. According to the new narrow economic perspective, the determination of those who deserve to be included within the Israeli society, no longer included motherhood and childcare work. In this context, traditional conceptions, which valued motherhood, became reshaped and subordinate to the worker's image: which was that of the ideal male worker. Against this standard, women were now measured, as Prime Minister Ariel Sharon said at the Caesarea conference: "When I look at the basis of our social-economic program, I see before me the working man, he who is working for his livelihood in uneasy conditions, who bears on his shoulders the economic burden. The Zionist revolution was based on this person and we need to return him to our society" (p. 2).

In the new political economy, old perceptions cherishing motherhood, defining it as an appreciated national aim were replaced, and mothers were evaluated mainly according to their economic value, and thus their ability to financially provide for themselves and for their family members. While in the past mothers' responsibility included the socialization of their children to become law-abiding citizens, they were now assigned a new role, dictated by the new values of the state: they were required to be modest, abstemious, and ready to work. Mothers were called upon to care for their children by following these new rules and joining the workforce.

In this way, a new definition of citizenship was created, redefining the criteria for deserved inclusion within Israeli society, devaluing motherhood, and subordinating it to values of productivity and participation in the workforce. An economic citizenship was established; a model of citizenship which is predicated on a male model of citizenship that links it to the labor market (see Kessler-Harris, 2001; Orloff, 1999). This model replaced the older social citizenship model which valued, among other things, women's contribution to society as mothers.

Employment was defined as a means to enhance the Israeli economy, ignoring questions of availability of work and the high rate of unemployment, and in effect transferring the responsibility for employment to the citizens. The unemployed, mainly single, mothers were blamed by a government spokesperson for sitting idly and refusing to look for jobs waiting for them. The government called upon them to look for work actively: "Do not say that there is no work, but make yourself a better worker, productive, efficient, responsible. Workers will bring work to places where there is no work." (http://www.netanyahu.org/xruecu.html).

Thus, during the twenty-first century, individuals in Israel are now evaluated for societal membership according to the work they do and how much they earn. This is grounded in the neo-liberal ideological move toward individualization which emphasized "self sufficiency and independence coupled to the market activation of all individuals and groups" (Hobson, 2003, p. 75). This created the ideological and practical framework within which the Israeli government turned away from its commitment to women as caregivers, exposing them, without protection, to the labor forces, and thus leading to the poverty and abuse of many women (Swirski, 2003).

Driven by the neo-liberal ideology and mentality, social policy in Israel further altered the relations between families, children, and the state. The family of certain social groups in the new regime is conceived as a problematic unit, a place which reproduces negative norms of dependency, nonproductivity, and exploitation (Ajzenstadt, 2009). In contrast to the family, the labor market is represented as an ideal site, enabling recovery and rebuilding people and even the entire community. The family institution which was idealized and regarded as being central to society in previous periods, has been redefined as a dangerous location which does not encourage its members to join the labor market where they would be productive, responsible, and able to care for themselves.

Finally, while children were considered by the Zionist ethos and during most of the twentieth century to be assets, symbolizing the future of the nation, in the twenty-first century social polices redefined children, especially those belonging to the lower socio-economic populations, as expensive and as obstacles to the integration of mothers into the workforce. Yitzhak Kadman, the Director of the National Council for the Child, questioned the new definition of the family in the official discourse, suggesting that the Israeli government envisioned a new society: "a society of families who include one child and a dog, committed to shares in the stock exchange market" (Labor, Welfare and Health Committee, Protocol No. 8. 31.3.2003).

The new regime, which encouraged the integration of mothers into the labor force, did not provide childcare or other family-friendly policies (see discussion in

Lewis & Campbell, 2007; Lewis, Knijn, Martin, & Ostner, 2008). Contradictory to the 1970s, the state did not take upon itself the responsibility for childcare while mothers worked outside the home. In addition, it did not create affordable arrangements to care for children during regular working hours. Single mothers, for example, who refuse to work in jobs requiring their presence between 7.30–8.00 and until 17.00 because their children are not cared for during the morning and evening hours, lose their eligibility for income support for two months (Lotan, 2007, p. 7). In this way caring for children has remained a private, family responsibility and mothers must obey the new rules of economic citizenship while simultaneously caring for their children without supportive state policies.

Current official discourse is economically oriented, taking precedence over other possible narratives and stripping the State of Israel of its traditional ideological orientations which have shaped its activities and discursive formations in relation to women, children, and families. Ehud Razaby, a member of the liberal Shinui party expressed this view: "people still think that Israel should be a welfare state ... in order to be a welfare state, you need to be strong, you need to have lots of financial resources. The existence of resources is the only condition for being a welfare state, it is simple, you do not need anything else" (Labor, Welfare and Health Committee, Protocol No. 8. 31.3.2003, p. 15). Attempting to re-shape the discussion in other terms, Kadman, the executive director of the Israeli National Council for the Child said: "the state of Israel is not about profit, it is not a profitable business" (Labor, Welfare and Health Committee, Protocol No. 8. 31.3.2003, p. 14). However, this counter discourse has had no impact on the way in which Israel now treats women, families, and children.

Concluding Remarks

Israeli society is currently located at a juncture in which old constructs of citizenship, femininity, and masculinity are being neglected and new concepts are being constructed. In the past, the welfare state in Israel, its discourses and ideological and cultural premises were closely linked to the mission of building the nation. Social policy programs served as instruments of state and nation building, including the absorption of individuals and groups. This ideology made motherhood the core relationship of normative social life and as long as they adhered to the core values of society and a commitment to fulfill their traditional roles, women were entitled to state benefits and protection.

Recent social policy has turned away from this approach and instead adopted a narrow perspective which measures social participation not in terms of individual contribution to nation building, but in economic terms, defined mainly by disassociation with welfare payments. Social policies developed relatively recently, as well as the dominant rationalities and practices, have drastically altered the relations between women, children, and families which were developed at the end of the nineteenth century and through most of the twentieth century.

The changing meaning of citizenship in general, and the various paths defined as required for the inclusion of women and children in Israeli society, in particular, indicates that citizenship is a "contextualized concept" (Siim, 2000, p. 1). It is both a status involving rights conferred on individuals and a practice involving responsibilities to the wider society. Gendered vocabularies of citizenship and their meanings vary according to social, political, and cultural context, reflecting different historical legacies. Moreover, citizenship is not a social status which is distinct from both political participation and economic dependence, and is practiced in both the public and private realms (see discussion in Prokhovnik, 1998). Between 1880 and 2008, the "sexual contract" (cf. Pateman, 1988) between women and the state has changed and new terms have been established which have been accompanied by new rationalities and mentalities which are redefining and reshaping citizenship. According to the new contract, new female duties were created, centering on work obligations as a central element of citizenship. It remains to be seen whether under the present model of citizenship, past social constructs will be totally ignored, or society adopts new modes of relations between women, children, and families, more similar to past modes.

References

Abramovitz, M. (2000). *Under attack, fighting back: Women and welfare in the United States.* New York: Monthly Review Press.

Achdut, N. (2007). The Program for the integration of single parents in the labor market: Resources and obstructions for the integration in the employment arena. *Social Security, 73,* 69–111 (Hebrew).

Ajzenstadt, M. (2001). The construction of juvenile delinquency in light of normality, Palestine 1922–1944. *Megamot, 41*(1–2), 71–96 (Hebrew).

Ajzenstadt, M. (2002). Crime, social control and the process of social classification: Juvenile delinquency/justice discourse in Israel, 1948–1970. *Social Problems, 49*(4), 585–604.

Ajzenstadt, M. (2009). Moral panic and Neo-Liberalism: The case of single mothers on welfare in Israel. *British Journal of Criminology, 49*(1), 68–87.

Ajzenstadt, M., & Cavaglion, G. (2002). The sexual body of the young Jew as an arena of ideological struggle: 1821–1948. *Symbolic Interaction, 25*(1), 93–116.

Ajzenstadt, M., & Gal, J. (2001). Appearances can be deceptive: Gender in the Israeli welfare state. *Social Politics: International Studies in Gender, State, and Society, 8*(3), 292–324.

Ajzenstadt, M., & Rosenhek, Z. (2000). Privatization and new modes of state intervention: The long-term care program in Israel. *Journal of Social Policy, 29*(2), 247–262.

Almogi, Y. (1969). Women labor is necessary for the market. *Labor and National Insurance, 22,* 130–131.

Azaryahu, S. ([1948] 1977). *The union of Hebrew women for equal rights in Eretz Israel: Chapters in the history of the women's movement of Eretz Israel.* Haifa: Women's Aid Fund.

Bar, H., & Markus, Y. (1977). *Day-care: A social service for the mother and her child: A survey of workers and consumers.* Jerusalem: Institute for Applied Social Research (Hebrew).

Becker, N., Abhasera, N., & Ziv, C. (2006). *Invisible workers in the public service: A report on violation of contractor's workers rights in government offices.* Jerusalem: Faculty of Law, Hebrew University of Jerusalem (Hebrew).

Ben-Porath, Y. (1986). Diversity in population and in the labor force. In Y. Ben-Porath (Ed.), *The Israeli economy: Maturing through crises* (pp. 153–170). Cambridge, MA: Harvard University Press.

Berkovitch, N. (1997). Motherhood as a national mission: The construction of womanhood in the legal discourse in Israel. *Women's Studies International Forum, 20,* 605–620.

Bernstein, D. (1981). 'Come to grow with us ...': The place of women labor power in the Israeli economic development. *Notebooks of Research and Critique, 7,* 5–36.

Bernstein, D. (1984). Conflict and protest in Israeli society: The case of the Black Panthers of Israel. *Youth and Society, 16,* 129–152.

Bernstein, D. (1992). Human being or housewife? The status of women in the Jewish working class family in Palestine of the 1920s and 1930s. In D. S. Bernstein (Ed.), *Pioneers and homemakers: Jewish women in pre-state Israel* (pp. 235–256). New York: SUNY Press.

Blau, J., & Abramovitz, M. (2004). *The dynamics of social welfare policy.* New York: Oxford University Press.

Central Bureau of Statistics. (2008). *International women's day.* Retrieved from http://www.cbs. gov.il/reader/newhodaot/hodaa_template.html?hodaa=200811035 (Hebrew).

Crompton, R. (2006). *Employment and the family: The reconfiguration of work and family life in contemporary societies.* New York: Cambridge University Press.

Dagan-Bozaglo, N. (2007). *The right to work: A legal and economic perspective.* Retrieved from http://www.adva.org/view.asp?lang=he&catID=452 (Hebrew).

Davidov, G. (2007). *Enforcing labor and employment laws: Lessons from public-sector sub-contracting in Israel.* Paper presented at the Law and Society Association conference, Berlin.

Doron, A. (1985). The Israeli welfare state at crossroads. *Journal of Social Policy, 14,* 513–525.

Doron, A. (2005). Thatcher: The Israeli version. In R. Rothental (Ed.), *The roots: A new discourse on nation and society* (pp. 256–274). Jerusalem: Keter (Hebrew).

Elbashan, Y. (2004). Access of justice of marginalized groups in Israel. *Allei-Mishapt, 3,* 497–530 (Hebrew).

Elboim-Dror, R. (1994). Gender in utopianism: The Zionist case. *History Workshop, 37,* 99–111.

Filc, D. (2005). The health business under Neo-Liberalism: The Israeli case. *Critical Social Policy, 25*(2), 180–197.

Firer, R. (1984). The rise and fall of pioneer myth. *Kivunim, 23,* 5–23 (Hebrew).

Fraser, N. (1994). After the family wage: Gender equity and the welfare state. *Political Theory, 22*(4), 591–618.

Gal, J., & Achdut, N. (2007). A safety net full of holes: Changing policy towards Israel's social assistance program. In A. Uri, G. John, & J. Katan (Eds.), *Formulating social policy in Israel* (pp. 59–100). Jerusalem: Taub Center for Social Policy Studies in Israel (Hebrew).

Gelber, Y. (1987). The consolidation of the Jewish community in Israel, 1936–1947. In M. Lissak, A. Shapira, & G. Cohen (Eds.), *The history of the Jewish community in Eretz-Israel since 1882 Vol. 2: The British Mandate* (pp. 303–463). Jerusalem: Bialik Institute.

Gillies, V. (2005). Meeting parents' needs? Discourses of 'support' and 'inclusion' in family policy. *Critical Social Policy, 25*(1), 70–90.

Gordon, D., & Eliav, T. (1992). *Single parent families 1991.* Jerusalem: National Insurance Institute, Research and Planning Authority.

Gordon, L. (1990). *Women, the state, and welfare.* Madison: University of Wisconsin Press.

Hacker, D. (2001). Single and married women in the law of Israel: A feminist perspective. *Feminist Legal Studies, 9,* 29–56.

Halperin-Kaddari, R., & Karo, I. (2007). *Women and family in Israel: Statistical bi-annual report.* Ramat-Gan, Israel: Faculty of Law, Bar-Ilan University (Hebrew).

Herzl, T. ([ca. 1902] 1960). *Altneuland (Old-Newland).* Haifa: Haifa Publishing.

Hirsch, D. (2008). Interpreters of occident to the awakening orient: The Jewish public health nurse in Mandate Palestine. *Comparative Studies in Society and History, 50*(1), 227–255.

Hobson, B. (2003). The individualised worker, the gender participatory and the gender equity models in Sweden. *Social policy and society, 3*(1), 75–83.

Interministerial Committee for the Encouragement of Female Labor. (1966). The report of the Interministerial Committee for the Encouragement of Female Labor. *Labor and National Insurance, 18,* 134–136.

Izraeli, D. N. (1992). Culture, policy, and women in dual-earner families in Israel. In S. D. Lewis, N. Izraeli, & H. Hootsmans (Eds.), *Dual-earner families: International perspectives* (pp. 19–46). London: Sage.

Katznelson-Rubatchov, R. (1947, July 11). *Oral evidence presented at public meetings of the United Nations Special Committee on Palestine.* Lake Success, New York. [Verbatim record of the 27th meeting (public)]. Supplement no. 11.

Kessler-Harris, A. (2001). *In pursuit of equity: Women, men, and the quest for economic citizenship in 20th-century America.* Oxford, UK: Oxford University Press.

Kohavi, D. (1964). The extension of labor for women. *Labor and National Insurance, 16,* 104–106.

Lahav, P. (1993). When the "palliative" only spoils things: The parliamentary debate on the equal rights law. *Zrmmim, 46–47,* 149–159 (Hebrew).

Lewis, J. (1992). Gender and the development of welfare regimes. *Journal of European Social Policy, 2*(3), 159–173.

Lewis, J., & Campbell, M. (2007). UK work/family balance policies and gender equality, 1997–2005. *Social Politics: International Studies in Gender, State & Society, 14*(1), 1–27.

Lewis, J., & Giullari, S. (2005). The adult worker model family, gender equality and care: The search for new policy principles and the possibilities and problems of a capabilities approach. *Economy and Society, 34*(1), 76–104.

Lewis, J., Knijn, T., Martin, C., & Ostner, I. (2008). Patterns of development in work/family reconciliation policies for parents in France, Germany, the Netherlands, and the UK in the 2000s. *Social Politics: International Studies in Gender, State and Society, 15*(3), 261–286.

Lissak, M. (1995). Immigration, absorption and society building in Israel during the first two decades (1918–1930). In M. Lissak, A. Shapira, & G. Cohen (Eds.), *The history of the Jewish community in Eretz-Israel since 1882, Vol. 2: The British Mandate* (pp. 173–302). Jerusalem: Bialik Institute.

Lissak, M. (1999). *The mass immigration in the fifties: The failure of the melting pot policy.* Jerusalem: The Bialik Institute.

Lotan, O. (2007). *Employment and poverty among single mothers.* Jerusalem: The Centre of Research and Information, The Knesset (Hebrew).

The Ministry of Industry, Trade and Labor. (2006). *Women in the labor market: 25 facts on women in Israel.* Jerusalem: The Ministry of Industry, Trade and Labor (Hebrew).

Nakar, Y. (2006). *Women in Israel 2001–2006.* The Knesset Information Services 2006 (Hebrew).

The National Insurance Institute of Israel. (2002). *Statistical quarterly, July–September.* Jerusalem: The National Insurance Institute of Israel.

Nitzan, J., & and Bichler, S. (2002). *The global political economy of Israel.* London: Pluto Press.

Nordau, M. (1955). *Zionist writings* (Vol. 1). Jerusalem: World Zionist Organization (Hebrew).

O'Connor, J. S. (1993). Gender class and citizenship in the comparative analysis of welfare states: Theoretical and methodological issues. *The British Journal of Sociology, 44*(3), 501–518.

O'Connor, J. S., Orloff, A. S., & Shaver, S. S. (1999). *States, markets, families, gender, liberalism and social policy in Australia, Canada, Great Britain and the United States.* Cambridge: Cambridge University Press.

Okun, B. S., Oliver, A. L., & Khait-Marelly, O. (2007). The public sector, family structure, and labor market behavior: Jewish mothers in Israel. *Work and Occupations, 34*(2), 174–204.

Orloff, A. (1999). Motherhood, work and welfare in the United States, Britain, Canada and Australia. In G. Steinmetz (Ed.), *State/culture: State formation after the cultural turn* (pp. 291–320). Ithaca: Cornell University Press.

Pateman, C. (1988). *The sexual contract.* Stanford: Stanford University Press.

Prokhovnik, R. (1998). Public and private citizenship: From gender invisibility to feminist inclusiveness. *Feminist Review, 60*(1), 80–104.

Raday, F. (1994). On equality. *Mishpatim, 24,* 241–281 (Hebrew).

Raday, F. (1999). The Insider-Outsider politics of labor-only contracting. *Comparative Labor Law and Policy Journal, 20,* 413–445.

Rapoport, T., & El-Or, T. (1997). Cultures of womanhood in Israel: Social agencies and gender production. *Women's Studies International Forum, 20*(5–6), 573–580.

Razin, A., & Sadka, E. (1993). *The economy of modern Israel: Malaise and promise*. Chicago: University of Chicago Press.

Rosenhek, Z. (2004). The Israeli welfare state crisis and the globalization process: Points of comparison. In M. Maor (Ed.), *State and community* (pp. 46–52). Jerusalem: The Hebrew University of Jerusalem, Magnes Press (Hebrew).

Sainsbury, D. (1994). Women's and men's social rights: Gendering dimensions of welfare states. In D. Sainsbury (Ed.), *Gendering welfare states* (pp. 150–169). London: Sage.

Sainsbury, D. (1999). *Gender and welfare state regimes*. Oxford: Oxford University Press.

Salzberger, L. (1995). *Socio-familial deprivation over time: The impact of accelerated social opportunity inputs on the mobility of socially deprived families in Jerusalem 1965–1975.* Jerusalem: Academon (Hebrew).

Shachak, I. (2003). *The economic distress of single mothers*. Jerusalem, Israel: Knesset Center of Research and Information (Hebrew).

Shafir, G., & Peled, Y. (2002). *Being Israeli: The dynamics of multiple citizenship*. Cambridge: Cambridge University Press.

Sheffer, N. (1999). *The Israel government policy in subsidizing daycare: Its implications for the work of women outside the home*. Position paper written for the Israel Women's Network. Jerusalem: Israel Women's Network.

Shilo, M. (2007). *The gender challenge: Women in the first immigration waves*. Tel-Aviv: The Kibbutz Hameuhad (Hebrew).

Siim, B. (2000). *Gender and citizenship*. Cambridge: Cambridge University Press.

Smooha, S. (1993). Class, communal and national gaps and democracy in Israel. In U. Ram (Ed.), *Israeli society: Critical perspective* (pp. 172–202). Breirot: Tel Aviv (Hebrew).

Steinberg, B. (1988). Education and integration in Israel: The first twenty years. *The Jewish Journal of Sociology, 30*(1), 17–36.

Steir, H. (1998). Short-term employment transitions of women in the Israeli labor force. *Industrial and Labor Relations Review, 51*, 269–281.

Steir, H., & Lewin-Epstein, N. (2000). Women's part-time employment and gender inequality in the family. *Journal of Family Issues, 21*(3), 390–410.

Steir, H., Lewin-Epstein, N., & Braun, M. (2001). Welfare regimes, family-supportive policies, and women's employment along the life-course. *American Journal of Sociology, 106*(6), 1731–1760.

Steir, H., & Yaish, M. (2008). The determinants of women's employment dynamics: The case of Israeli women. *European Sociological Review, 24*(3), 363–377.

Stoler-Liss, S. (2003). This is how I would grow a Zionist baby: The construction of the Israeli baby and mother through training books to parents. *Studies in the Establishment of Israel, 13*, 277–293.

Swirski, B. (2003). A gendered perspective on the Social Security Net: Income support allowance. Tel Aviv: Adva Center – Information on Equality and Social Justice in Israel (Hebrew).

Swirski, S., & Bernstein, D. (1981). Who worked at what, for whom, and in return for what? Economic development in Israel and the evolution of the division of labor. *Notebooks for Theory and Critique, 4*, 5–66 (Hebrew).

Swirski, S., Kraus, V., Konor-Atias, E., & Herbst, A. (2002). Mothers in Israel. *Information on Equality, 12*. Retrieved from http://www.adva.org (Hebrew).

Tagar, M. (2006). *Working without honor: Workers' rights and their abuse. A report of the Association for Human Rights on the occasion of International Human Rights Day*. Retrieved from http://www.acri.org.il/hebrew-acri/engine/story.asp?id=1429 (Hebrew).

Tahon, H. (1937). Social work in neighborhood stations. *News of Social Work in Eretz Israel, 2*, 173–176 (Hebrew).

Tamir, T. (2007). *Women in Israel: Between theory and reality*. Ramat Gan: Women Lobby in Israel.

Voet, R. (1998). *Feminism and citizenship*. London: Sage.

Warzberger, R. (2002). *Employment in manpower agencies*. Jerusalem, Israel: Knesset Center of Research and Information (Hebrew).

Warzberger, R. (2003). *The impact on the national insurance rights of single mothers following the cuts in the 2003 budget*. Jerusalem: Israel: Knesset Center of Research and Information (Hebrew).

Western, B. (1999). *Between class and market: Postwar unionization in the capitalist democracies*. Princeton: Princeton University Press.

Williams, F. (1995). Race/ethnicity, gender, and class in welfare states: A framework for comparative analysis. *Social Politics, 2*(2), 127–159.

Yaish, M., & Kraus, V. (2003). The consequences of economic restructuring for the gender earnings gap in Israel, 1972–1995. *Work Employment and Society, 17*(1), 5–28.

Yuval-Davis, N. (1993). Gender and nation. *Ethnic and Racial Studies, 16*(4), 621–632.

Gender, Family and Children at the Crossroads of Social Policy Reform in Turkey: Alternating Between Familialism and Individualism

Azer Kılıç

Introduction

In the last decade Turkey has undergone a process of reform in the field of social policy. This reform reached its most decisive and controversial phase with recent legislation regarding the Turkish social insurance and healthcare system. Until recently Turkey's welfare policies have relied largely on the model of the male-breadwinner family both as a source and a normative framework of welfare provision.

The recent reform process shows changes in this policy approach. First of all there is a move toward the individualization of some benefits that formerly, based on the principle of familial dependency, were granted to women and children through male family members. In addition, some gender-differentiated entitlements have been neutralized. Despite the introduction and/or extension of some benefits in this route, the overall trend implies more reliance on the market. Simultaneously, in certain areas of social policy, there has been an emphasis on using the family unit to decrease state responsibility. This chapter argues that an underlying rationality of neo-liberalism unifies these seemingly contradictory trends.

The prospects and limits of Turkish welfare reforms in terms of gender, family, and children are examined below. First, the Turkish welfare system and its recent reform are outlined. Then policy issues in Turkey's social protection system as it relates to gender, family, and children are elaborated upon. Next, major changes in protective legislation and recent trends in the labor market, especially in terms of female employment, are clarified. Finally, the conclusion presents an overall evaluation of the changing nature of the Turkish welfare system.

A. Kılıç (✉)
Max Planck Institute for the Study of Societies, Cologne, Germany
e-mail: azerkilic@gmail.com

The author gratefully acknowledges the support of the Boğaziçi University Social Policy Forum for the preparation of this article.

M. Ajzenstadt, J. Gal (eds.), *Children, Gender and Families in Mediterranean Welfare States*, Children's Well-Being: Indicators and Research 2, DOI 10.1007/978-90-481-8842-0_8, © Springer Science+Business Media B.V. 2010

The Turkish Welfare System and Its Ongoing Reform

With roots dating back to the late Ottoman era, the Turkish welfare system was developed by and large following World War II. Historically, the system relied mainly on a multi-fragmented, corporatist social security system in which separate insurance schemes were established for different occupational categories.[1] Each occupational category has different rules and benefits and is financed by contributions from the insured and their employer. The system, parallel to the labor market structure of the time, was established around a normative model of the family in which men were the principal breadwinners and women were responsible for domestic work including child care. Because of the underdevelopment of the social-assistance pillar of the system and the nature of the labor market in which self-employment, unpaid family work, and informal employment practices are central, the formal welfare system inadequately provides social protection to large sectors of the population. As a result, the system has been complemented by informal mechanisms like family and kinship solidarity as well as clientalistic relationships with the political authorities (Buğra & Keyder, 2006).

In the post-1980 period, market-oriented economic policies and the changing rural and urban structures had negative effects on informal social support mechanisms and the labor market. This resulted in an increased incapacity to combat rising risks and emerging forms of poverty (Buğra, 2007b). Accordingly, a number of social assistance schemes were introduced. The most important scheme is the Social Cooperation and Solidarity Encouragement Fund (1986), an umbrella organization covering over 900 local foundations and providing emergency relief, mostly in kind, to the poor. The establishment of the Fund, now a Directorate (SYDGM; General Directorate of Social Cooperation and Solidarity), indicated an implicit admission that the family was increasingly inadequate in its de facto role of welfare provision (ibid.). Another initiative is the Green Card scheme (1992) which provides healthcare for the uninsured poor on the basis of a means-test. Since then, initiatives for poverty alleviation have been dominated by an understanding of traditional charity, public–private–voluntary sector partnerships, and workfare (i.e., "new welfare governance") (Buğra, 2007b; Savaşkan, 2007; cf. Jessop, 1999; Bode, 2006).

Meanwhile, the ongoing socio-economic problems, mainly triggered by the economic crises of 2001, increased demands for reform of the social protection system. The fiscal crises of the social security system due to the high ratio of passive recipients to active contributors, the arbitrary use of social insurance funds by the state, who later attempted to cover up resulting deficits by using the public budget, and commitments to stand-by agreements with the International Monetary Fund (IMF) were stated as the major reasons for the reform. Other factors influential in this process include the legislative harmonization process for European Union (EU)

---

[1] Major social security institutions include: the Social Insurance Institution (SSK) for workers founded in 1945, the Retirement Chest (ES) for civil servants founded in 1949 and Bağ-Kur for the self-employed founded in 1971.

membership, the reform proposals regarding healthcare and retirement by the World Bank and national business circles, societal and labor-union opposition to such reform proposals, and the conservative liberal approach of the governing Justice and Development Party (*Adalet ve Kalkınma Partisi* – AKP).

The process mainly started with the reform of retirement schemes in 1999. This reform increased minimum age thresholds and premium payment requirements and culminated in the Social Insurances and General Health Insurance Law (No. 5489) of April 2006. The 2006 legislation planned a structural transformation of the existing social insurance schemes and the healthcare system, aiming at unifying the formerly separate insurance schemes into a single system.[2] The reform bill attempted to equalize norms and standards for all the insured persons and oblige the state to contribute to the system as well. According to the existing system, the minimum retirement age was 58 for women and 60 for men, while the minimum premium requirements were 7,000 days for workers and 9,000 days for civil servants and the self-employed. The reform of 2006 aimed to maintain these retirement ages until 2036, followed by a gradual equalization until 2048, when the minimum retirement age for both men and women would rise to 65 and the minimum premium requirement would be 9,000 days. Moreover, the reform planned changes in the pension calculation method in order to decrease the amount of future pensions.

In December of 2006, just before the law was to be implemented, some of its provisions were annulled by the Turkish Constitutional Court in order to protect the "acquired rights" of civil servants. This move was interpreted as state paternalism for civil servants and neo-liberal policies for workers (Çelik, 2007). The implementation of the law was postponed by the government until 2008. While the unification of the insurance schemes would increase institutional efficiency and terminate the hierarchy of benefits among the insured, the fact that this equalization of retirement rules also resulted in an erosion of social rights caused fierce labor opposition. Hence, the ratification of Bill 5754 was accompanied by intense controversy including parliamentary opposition by other parties and nationwide demonstrations by several labor unions, the Chamber of Doctors, and feminist organizations against the bill and the government's proposal for its amendment. After negotiations with the Labor Platform, the network of labor unions unified against the reform, the government responded to some demands, though not without a further erosion of social rights in other areas.

As a result of these negotiations the minimum premium requirement for workers was agreed to be 7,200 days, the age thresholds were kept as in the reform bill and pension amounts were further decreased. As a solution to the decision of the

---

[2] In addition to social insurance and healthcare, the reform package originally included a draft proposal for Social Assistances and Non-Contributory Payments. This proposal has not been brought to the parliament or sufficiently debated. In fact, it is not certain if the full draft proposal will ever be taken to parliament. The proposal included policies like the introduction of child and disability allowances, improving work prospects for assistance recipients, and minimum income support. It also planned to bring social assistance and social security arrangements within the same administrative framework.

Constitutional Court, civil servants who were insured before the reform were subject
to the original regulations and those who were insured after the reform were subject
to the new rules. Thus, despite fierce opposition, in April 2008 amendment bill no.
5754 was finally passed in the parliament.

The reform also proposed a system of universal health insurance, financed by
compulsory premiums on behalf of citizens earning above the poverty line.[3] On
the basis of a means-test, the state will pay healthcare premiums for those below
the poverty line, calculated as less than one third of the minimum income for each
individual in a household. Failure to pay the required premium, even if just for a
certain period of time, will result in restriction of access to health services, except
in cases of emergency.

However, premium collection is complicated, considering the fact that informal employment constitutes half of the labor force (World Bank, 2006). While
some informally employed persons have access to healthcare as dependents of an
insured family member, more than one-third of the total population (about 36%) are
not covered by any health insurance, including the Green Card program (World
Bank & SIS, 2005).[4] In such an environment, the move from the current fragmented healthcare system to a universal healthcare system, providing coverage to
the entire population, seems vital. However, the conflict between trends of privatization and marketization of service provision on the one hand, and demands for
increased contribution from the public budget (as demanded by several labor unions
and the Chamber of Doctors), or the financing of the system mainly by taxes (as
demanded by some academics and feminists) on the other hand, has caused significant controversy regarding the method of financing such a system. Despite this
tension, the major principles of the healthcare system proposed by the reform were
maintained.

---

[3]The dependents of the insured person – an uninsured spouse, children under 18 (or 25, depending
on educational and marital status), and parents who are cared for by the insured – will benefit
from the services as a part of his/her insurance. According to this system, retirees and survivor
pensioners would be exempt from paying premiums. However, all persons would be obliged to pay
user fees for healthcare services and some medicine costs.

[4]The provision and financing of the existing healthcare system is quite fragmented, with both public and private providers and financiers. However, the public sector predominates both in provision
and financing. Eighty-nine percent of the population (including repeated registers) are insured by
the three main insurance schemes while the Green Card program covers about 15.3% of the population (TÜSİAD, 2004). Yet, in practice there is a significant discrepancy between the percentage
of the population insured and access to healthcare in practice. The main factors preventing access
to healthcare are informal and irregular forms of employment, ineligibility for the Green Card program and premium debts to Bağ-Kur (there is no obligation for those insured under Bağ-Kur to
register for healthcare insurance). For instance, many of the insured who are self-employed cannot
regularly pay the monthly premium to Bağ-Kur. As of 2006, 60% of these insured persons were not
eligible for healthcare insurance due to premium debts. This fact illustrates the risks of a healthcare
reform based on required premium payments (Üstündağ & Yoltar, 2007, p.74).

The Social Protection System: From Familialism to Individualism?

While certain aspects of the Turkish social protection system have remained unchanged, other aspects have undergone significant transformation as a result of recent reforms. By looking at the historical development of the system from the perspective of gender, family, and children, a shift, although inconsistent, from familialism towards individualism is evident. Before examining examples of this shift, the two concepts must be clarified.

Familialism is commonly used to refer to the assignment of certain welfare responsibilities to the family (Esping-Anderson, 2006). This can be in the form of the de facto centrality of family solidarity in welfare provision even in the absence of formal responsibilities placed on the family unit (Leon, 2002). On the other hand, a specific familial model can also provide a normative framework for a formal social protection system. Here familialist social policies would be those which "assume and reinforce an ideal of the family," either as an end in itself or as a means to some other nonfamilial goal (Michel, 2000). Such policies take into account assumptions about gender roles and the division of labor, and family status is a central factor in determining entitlements. A common example are social insurance schemes which rely on a male-breadwinner family model, where women and children are entitled to derived benefits as dependents of the insured male heads of their family and women are discouraged from working.

On the other hand, in less familialistic systems benefits are granted to persons independent of familial status. Entitlements can be based on labor market status and the contributions of the individual recipients. In these systems women are encouraged to work. However, this does not always happen through measures that take into account their domestic responsibilities and enable work (Leon, 2002). Relevant examples include systems that formally support gender equality while risking the subjugation of women to the ideal of the male worker without domestic responsibilities. Alternatively, entitlements can be based on citizenship status and involve universal social rights granted to individuals, including children, furthering both defamilialization and decommodification (Sainsbury, 1996). Furthermore, means-tested noncontributory schemes for social assistance can operate through individualized eligibility criteria, although the socio-economic situation of the household as a whole is usually taken into account. As discussed below, the nature of the recent social policy reform process in Turkey oscillates between the two poles of familialism and individualism.

Social Insurance and Healthcare

Traditionally, Turkey's social protection system has been highly familialistic; the family has provided both an informal mechanism and a formal normative framework for welfare provision. According to this familial model, men are the principle breadwinners and women are responsible for care and housekeeping. Women are not considered a central component of the labor force and those women who do participate in the labor market are encouraged to leave. Hence, women are integrated into the social security system mainly as dependents of their insured family members – either as wives, daughters, or mothers – and granted benefits like healthcare on the basis of familial status.[5] The assumption of the male-breadwinner familial model is most apparent through the entitlement of dependent children to healthcare: the daughters of insured persons have been entitled to healthcare regardless of age as long as they are not married or formally employed. On the other hand, sons are subjected to age limits and exempt from this requirement only in case of disability or destitution.

Furthermore, in the case of the death of male heads of family, the state has assumed the burden of responsibility for wives and children through survivor pensions until they become employed or (re)married. In the case of divorce and unemployment, survivor wives and daughters have been re-entitled to benefits, yet were simultaneously encouraged to (re)marry via a lump sum payment of pensions. When the survivor schemes were established in the 1940s reasons stated as the basis for this gender-differentiated treatment included a lack of employment opportunities for women and the prevalence of a family structure which prevented the participation of women in the labor market. In addition, there existed a paternalistic state rhetoric which claimed that the state protected "destitute" women with these schemes. As for men, widowers were subjected to means-tests in order to be eligible for support since they were expected to be the breadwinner and survivor sons were entitled to benefits only until a certain age. As a result of such assumptions about gender roles, survivor sons, entitled to pensions in case of disability, were not subject to any other condition, whereas the pensions of disabled daughters were terminated in case of marriage. This fact indicates that such gender-differentiated treatment is based on an assumption of women's dependency on a male-headed family as opposed to a positive discrimination policy to compensate disadvantages.

Reform initiatives have changed certain aspects of this long-lasting policy. First of all, in the mid-1980s policy changes began to equalize the conditions for surviving spouses making marital status the main requirement. The 2006 reform was intended to complete this equalization of survivor spouses by extending marriage allowances to male survivors in addition to female. However, in order to prevent the decrease of marriage allowances for survivor daughters, negotiations between the government and the labor platform concluded with the amendment bill of 2008

---

[5]For a more detailed discussion of the gender dimension of Turkey's social security system from both historical and contemporary perspectives, see Kılıç (2008a, 2008b). I should note that women and men are of course not homogenous groups; however, here I aim to outline such abstract categories as embodied in the social policy legislation and discourse and discuss their gendered implications for the majority of women, who are economically more vulnerable to social risks. On the other hand, one can notice that such a gendered social policy environment does not necessarily mean favoring men, either.

which terminated marriage allowances for all survivor spouses.[6] While the gendered treatment of orphans is still maintained,[7] the overall trend of gender-neutralization may signal a move from the ideal of the "male-breadwinner" towards a model of "universal breadwinner."[8]

The reform in the healthcare system shows a further step in the gender-neutralization of welfare benefits. This reform cancelled the entitlement of dependent daughters to lifelong health insurance by limiting their entitlement to 25 years of age depending on their educational and marital status and obligating them to pay healthcare premiums. Factions in the parliament have opposed this change stating that it deprives daughters of their "acquired rights" and claiming that by the age of 25 most women are not economically independent. Through public demonstrations and recommending alternative proposals, the Women's Platform for Social Rights, which brought together over 80 women's organizations against the bill, demanded free healthcare for all women independently of their fathers and husbands. Women argued that the reform increased their dependency on family and marriage and ignored domestic unpaid labor. Following this opposition, a transitional article was added to the amendment which maintained the acquired rights of daughters who had been entitled to healthcare before the reform, until they joined the work force or married.

Despite the fact that the family unit remains the recipient of healthcare insurance, this reform also signals a move from familialism to individualism in two ways. First of all, the reform introduced a noncontributory scheme for children under 18 years of age which prevents the dependence of children on both their family and the market for health insurance. This is particularly significant in light of the high rate of child poverty in Turkey; 34% of children under the age of 15 live below the poverty line (Yakut-Çakar & Buğra, 2007). Secondly, a contributory scheme was introduced for the single, formally unemployed women over 18 who would have benefited from health services thanks to their parents in the former system. This new policy relates to women as economically independent despite the low rates of female employment.

Retirement schemes were originally established around a similar set of ideals and assumptions regarding women. Working women were encouraged to return home and perform their familial duties through incentives of early retirement, after the

---

[6]The 2006 reform granted survivor sons, as well as daughters, marriage allowances. However, during the amendment process the government declared that this was a technical fault due to the fact that survivor sons' pensions are not terminated before they formally end as a result of marriage.

[7]Orphans are treated differently according to gender in all cases except for a 2003 reform which extended the disability pension to survivor females.

[8]Changes to Turkish civil law follow a parallel trend. The Civil Law of 1926, which was in force until the Law of 2001, relied on the male breadwinner family model, explicitly considering the husband the head of the family responsible for maintenance of the household, while regarding the wife as the housekeeper and subject to permission from her husband in order to work. In 1990 the provision regarding permission for work was annulled by the Constitutional Court and the rest was changed by the Civil Law of 2001, which ended the attributed roles of family head, maintenance and care and refers to the shared contributions of spouses reflected by their capability.

admittedly tiresome years of working a "double shift," one shift outside the house and one shift in the house. In addition, in the case of termination of work due to marriage, women received benefits such as repayment of premiums and severance pay. However, according to the 2006 reform the current retirement policy will be maintained until the year 2036, and then a gradual equalization of the genders will be realized by 2048, when the minimum retirement age for both sexes will rise to 65.

Working women and feminists opposed this reform as well. First of all, a high minimum retirement threshold of this nature is problematic considering the fact that female employment is more interrupted as a result of maternal and domestic responsibilities. In addition, the Women's Platform supported early retirement for working women until the problem of the double shift can be solved through equal sharing of domestic responsibilities at home and the expansion of public services for child and elderly care. Only then can women be treated the same as men. In spite of this opposition, the reform remained unchanged and the formal equalization of retirement schemes for both genders resulted in an erosion of women's rights. Not only was the retirement age increased for both women and men without implementing effective policies to reconcile work and family life, there have also been regressive attempts regarding child care services for working women (which will be explored below).

Social Assistance and Services

While historically the social assistance pillar of the Turkish welfare system has largely been neglected, in the post-1980 period some important mechanisms were developed as a response to increasing poverty. Implementation of social assistance initiatives increased specifically in the last few years with the family as an important normative framework. This is reflected in the AKP government rhetoric which often attributes society's ability to withstand harsh economic problems to its strong family structure. The AKP program also includes a family-centered social policy approach which encourages adult children to care for their elderly parents and reinforces the central role of the family in the rehabilitation of children in need of protection (AKP, 2001).

"Back to the Family" is an example of a program aimed to realize this goal. This program seeks to send children who are under institutional care by Social Services and the Children Protection Agency, mostly due to economic reasons, back to their families by providing monetary assistance to their immediate family (or extended family if immediate family does not exist) who remove their children from institutional care. In cases where this is not possible, the program encourages foster care and even adoption over institutional care (Yazıcı, 2007). In addition to the emphasis on family values, this project has been justified with reasons regarding economic efficiency. A similar policy to support home-based care has been applied to the care of the disabled as well. These policies in effect shift the burden of care from the state to the family, and particularly to women, who provide a significant source of unpaid labor. This exacerbates the effects of the already extremely low level of public spending on family benefits such as child allowances, nurseries, and preschool programs.

Conversely, the recent introduction of the Conditional Cash Transfer (CCT) program is a positive step against child poverty. CCT benefits are administered by SYDGM, initially in connection with the Social Risk Mitigation project of the World Bank, following the economic crises of 2001. This program has been implemented in varied forms throughout the developing world since the 1990s and been fully operational nationwide in Turkey since 2004. The program provides social assistance for the poorest 6% of the population conditional on the improved use of basic health and education services, targeting mainly the families that are not under social security coverage. The monetary allowance is provided to mothers and conditional on giving birth at a hospital (for those who are pregnant), regular check-ups including complete vaccination for children aged 0–6, and regular school attendance (primary and secondary levels). Although the amount of the CCT benefit is very small,[9] assessments show that the program has increased full-immunization rates and school attendance, especially by girls (Yakut-Çakar & Buğra, 2007). These benefits are critical in light of the fact that 43% of Turkish children have incomplete immunizations (ibid.) and the combined gross enrollment ratio for primary, secondary, and tertiary education is 68.7% for the total school age population and 64% for the female population (UNDP, 2007).

The gendered implications of the CCT program, however, seem somewhat complex. The fact that the cash is directly paid to mothers may have a positive impact on their empowerment within the household and that the amount is higher for girls seems appropriate in encouraging otherwise low female schooling. Yet, the fact that the responsibility to realize the principal conditions is given mainly to mothers reinforces the traditional gendered division of labor for care work.[10] This further reliance on female "voluntary" labor may also relate to the shift from the socialization of primary health services to the family medicine system, which is a pilot project underway, as an important component of the Transformation in Health Program.[11] In the former system, midwives from local health posts used to work in the field, paying visits to houses and hence facilitating the accessibility of preventive

---

[9]The amount of cash transfers varies according to the number, gender, age, and the educational level of children. In 2008, the amount given for primary school children was 20 YTL for boys and 25 YTL for girls and approximately 80% higher for the secondary school children (note that the minimum net wage was 435 YTL, which was about 228€). The allowances are granted for 9 months a year. See SYDGM (2008).

[10]Similar poverty relief programs elsewhere in the world seem to be working in the same gendered way, relying on women's unpaid labor for the functioning and success of those programs. For examples from Latin America, see Molyneux (2007) and Ewig (2006).

[11]For a detailed analysis of the transformation of the healthcare system see Ağartan (2005) and Günal (2007).

and curative basic services[12]; however, with the new system these services are to be accessed through family doctors in the public health centers. Thereby, the overall trend places an additional burden on poor women, assuming they are able and free to care for family members within and outside home.

Protective Legislation and Recent Trends in the Labor Market

Labor market policies historically reflected similar assumptions regarding gender roles and the family. Accordingly, men were regarded as the principal source of labor, whereas women were not regarded as an important component of the workforce and policy incentives encouraged women to return home. As of 2006, the participation rate of women in the workforce was 26.6% and decreased to 19.9% in urban areas (TÜİK, 2007). While female labor in the agricultural sector is mostly in the form of unpaid labor (around two-thirds), in the nonagricultural sector women's labor conditions are generally characterized by low-paid, nonskilled, labor-intensive occupations, which have the connotation of "female jobs." Furthermore, despite equal compensation laws for working women, women's salaries are usually less than those of men for equivalent work.[13] This fact is commonly justified by the assumption that women contribute to a male-headed family and thus, their income is a mere supplement to the family budget (Ecevit, 1998).

The dominance of a familialist approach appears to be the central reason for the low rate of female employment. Social norms regarding gender roles consider care and housekeeping as principally female responsibilities. According to household surveys, about two-thirds of women who did not participate in the labor force in 2006 state their preoccupation with housework as the major reason for their nonparticipation (TÜİK, 2007). Because of the lack of formal measures to reconcile work and family responsibilities, working women who leave the workforce also do so as a result of familial reasons (marriage, demand of the husband, child birth, and care of a child, the sick, or the elderly). Women who remain in the workforce rely mostly on female relatives to assume their domestic responsibilities.

In this case the recent reform process offers both positive and negative steps in the attempt to reconcile the responsibilities of both work and family. First of all, in 2003 as a commitment of Turkey's national program for the adoption of the EU

---

[12]Through home-visits, midwives monitor the health of pregnant women and their babies in the area they cover. During these visits, they can offer information on mother and child health, nutrition, first aid, prevention of diseases as well as providing primary-level care, vaccination, and family planning services.

[13]Monthly earnings of males are higher than those of females, in both public and private sectors, irrespective of educational status and economic branch of activity and this difference widens in the private sector (Toksöz, 2007). On average, women earn 78–83% of what men do (World Bank, 2006).

Acquis Communautaire,[14] paid maternity leave was increased from 12 to 16 weeks. In addition, the 2006 reform proposed extending the breast-feeding allowance to all insured persons (the ES and the Bağ-Kur did not include such a benefit formerly) for a period of 6 months in addition to incorporating maternity insurance into Bağ-Kur. Yet, with the 2008 amendment the breast-feeding allowance was decreased to 1 month.

Another commitment of the national program relates to parental leave. The agenda of the previous parliament included a draft law which defined the parental leave right for civil servants and workers. The draft law became void as a result of parliamentary elections, but it is likely to appear on the national agenda again, as this has been signaled by the government. According to this draft law, civil servants and workers (both male and female) are to be eligible for up to 12 months of unpaid parental leave following paid maternity leave. Such a shift from maternal leave to parental leave is an important step in the process of reconciling work and family life and in transforming the gendered division of labor at home and in the labor market. This policy allows responsibilities to be shared equally within the family and challenges employers' preference of men over women by leveling the amount of leave each is permitted to take. However, the result of similar policies in European countries show that men are unlikely to take leave unless it is paid and depending on the nature of the leave policy it may actually promote women's exit from the workforce (Bruning & Plantenga, 1999; Lewis & Giullari, 2005). Therefore, implementation of social policies for the provision of child care services and the reorganization of the labor market are also necessary.

However, the AKP government, given its recent legislation of law no. 5763, does not appear to intend to resolve these needs in the field of child care services. This law terminates the responsibility of both public and private employers of more than 150 women to provide day nurseries and breast-feeding rooms. The government first proposed granting cash benefits to working women to individually choose a child care provider. However, due to the high costs of this alternative, the AKP ultimately gave employers the option to purchase child care services from the market. This legislative package also includes a premium deduction for working women and young workers in an effort to increase their employment.

Another important change that occurred in 2003 was the cancellation of the long-standing prohibition against female industrial night-workers. Now only those younger than 18 are prohibited from industrial night-work. The cancellation of this prohibition might seem like a positive step in increasing the participation of women in the workforce. However, studies indicate that such an erosion of protective legislation may be less associated with giving "free choice" to women and more related to the deregulation of the labor market (Lewis & Davies, 1991).

---

[14]The term refers to the entire body of European laws, which must be adopted and implemented by the candidate countries to be allowed to join the EU. For the accession negotiations with Turkey, the *acquis* has been divided into 35 chapters, with a special chapter on social policy and employment as well. For an evaluation of the Turkish accession to the EU from a social policy perspective, see Manning (2007).

When taking into consideration the retirement reform, which institutes a later retirement age for working women as well as men, it is possible to view these changes as encouraging female employment as opposed to the former policy of encouraging working women to return home. However, the lack of public services for care, projects like "Back to the Home" regarding children, disabled, and the elderly and a new pro-natalist rhetoric (evident in the Prime Minister's recurring statements requesting Turkish women to bear at least three children in order to make up for Turkey's aging population) contradict policies that encourage female participation in the workforce.

Recent trends in the labor market and employment policies appear to present a resolution to this dilemma. While it is hard to speak of a well-developed policy on women's employment, entrepreneurship has been one of the most promoted strategies in the last two decades to increase female labor force participation and to combat poverty (Ecevit, 2007), despite the fact that poverty is most widespread among self-employed women (SPF, 2007: 13). Micro-finance has been one significant instrument for encouraging women into entrepreneurship and a resolution for the above-mentioned dilemma. Employment positions created through micro-credit, generally in traditionally "female occupations" such as carpet weaving and lacework, mostly function like other informal home-based work by reconciling work and family responsibilities in a gender-biased way. Such occupations provide the flexible work schedule necessary for women to fulfill their domestic responsibilities and, as they are located within the home or in female-dominated environments, encourage male consent when needed (Dedeoğlu, 2000). However, these occupations provide no social security benefits. Some of the practices that help women become micro-entrepreneurs actually result in the production of goods below normal market prices. This is the case of NGO workshops bringing women micro-entrepreneurs together (Buğra, 2007a).

In addition, the 2007 law no. 5588 on income tax regarded home-based working women as "independent own-account producers," though in actuality most are "dependent subcontract workers" (cf. Carr, Chen, & Tate, 2000). Within the new social protection system, this law prevents these women from claiming social security both as home workers and as formally unemployed dependents of the insured. Again this reflects a perception of women as small entrepreneurs as opposed to wage and salary earners. In the end, it seems that unjust gender order and neo-liberal policies go hand in hand.

Conclusion

Historically, the family unit has been an important institution and normative framework of service provision in the Turkish welfare state. Women and children were granted benefits, such as healthcare, under the assumption that they were dependents within a male breadwinner family. Accordingly, working women were expected to leave the labor market after marriage. This was encouraged by the absence of sufficient support services for working women with domestic responsibilities. However, the recent reform process indicates some changes in this family-centered approach to social policy.

Recently there has been a move toward the individualization of some benefits which were formerly granted to women and children as dependents, and the neutralization of some of the formerly gender-differentiated entitlements. In the process there has also been an introduction of a number of new entitlements and the extension of some existing benefits. Universal healthcare without a premium for children is the most significant step in this direction, furthering both defamilialization and decommodification.

However, other changes imply an increased reliance on the market. This is evident in the increase of the minimum retirement age to 65 for both men and women and the termination of the healthcare benefits for women over 18 on the basis of dependency. This type of policy relates to women as economically independent despite the fact that they have not actually integrated into the labor market and therefore places many women in an increasingly vulnerable position. Reforms in policies regarding night work, retirement, and premium deduction, as they relate to women, indicate that there has been a shift towards a policy of encouraging female employment. However, these reforms do not take into account domestic responsibilities that largely fall on women. Thus, formal policies to reconcile the responsibilities of family and work are necessary.

On the other hand, in certain policy areas the family has been used as a way to decrease state responsibility to social welfare. The lack of public services to assist with care indicates that the burden of unpaid care work on women seems unlikely to diminish soon. Some recent trends in the labor market do offer a means to reconcile the responsibilities of family and work. Home-based occupations, including both subcontracted and micro-credit jobs, help women tackle the "double shift" by allowing them to perform their work duties without disrupting the established gender division of domestic work which places the burden of this work on their shoulders. These trends also further the gender bias of the labor market and the existing social security structure. In this way neo-liberal and neo-conservative policies complement one another.

References

Ağartan, T. (2005). *Health sector reform in Turkey: Old policies new politics*. Paper presented at the 2005 ESPANET Young Researchers Workshop (July). Retrieved from http://www.cevipof.msh-paris.fr/rencontres/jours/200509-ante/palier/clegg/YR_papers/Agartan.pdf

AKP. (2001). Retrieved from http://www.akparti.org.tr/program.pdf

Bode, I. (2006). Disorganized welfare mixes: Voluntary agencies and new governance regimes in Western Europe. *Journal of European Social Policy, 16*(4), 346–359.

Bruning, G., & Plantenga, J. (1999). Parental leave and equal opportunities: Experiences in eight European countries. *Journal of European Social Policy, 9*(3), 195–209.

Buğra, A. (2007a). AKP döneminde sosyal politika ve vatandaşlık. *Toplum ve Bilim, 108*, 143–166.

Buğra, A. (2007b). Poverty and citizenship: An overview of the social-policy environment in republican Turkey. *International Journal of Middle East Studies*, *39*, 27–46.

Buğra, A., & Keyder, Ç. (2006). Turkish welfare regime in transformation. *Journal of European Social Policy*, *16*(3), 211–228.

Carr, M., Chen, M. A., & Tate, J. (2000). Globalization and home-based workers. *Feminist Economics*, *6*(3), 123–142.

Çelik, A. (2007). Sosyal güvenlik taarruzunda mola. *Birikim*, *213*, 8–12.

Dedeoğlu, S. (2000). Toplumsal cinsiyet rolleri açısından Türkiye'de aile ve kadın emeği. *Toplum ve Bilim*, *86*, 139–170.

Ecevit, Y. (1998). Türkiye'de ücretli kadın emeğinin toplumsal cinsiyet temelinde analizi. In A. B. Hacımirzaoğlu (Ed.), *75 yılda kadınlar ve erkekler* (pp. 267–284). Istanbul: Tarih Vakfı.

Ecevit, Y. (2007). *A critical approach to women entrepreneurship in Turkey*. Ankara: International Labor Office.

Esping-Anderson, G. (2006). Toplumsal riskler ve refah devletleri. In A. Buğra & Ç. Keyder (Eds.), *Sosyal politika yazıları* (pp. 33–54). Istanbul: İletişim.

Ewig, C. (2006). Global processes, local consequences: Gender equity and health sector reform in Peru. *Social Politics*, *13*(3), 427–455.

Günal, A. (2007). *Health and citizenship in republican Turkey: An analysis of the socialization of health services in the republican historical context*. Ph.D. dissertation, Boğaziçi University.

Jessop, B. (1999). The changing governance of welfare: Recent trends in its primary functions, scale and mode of cooperation. *Social Policy & Administration*, *33*(4), 348–359.

Kılıç, A. (2008a). Continuity and change in social policy approaches toward women. *New Perspectives on Turkey*, *38*(Spring), 135–158.

Kılıç, A. (2008b). The gender dimension of social policy reform in Turkey: Towards equal citizenship? *Social Policy & Administration*, *42*(5), 487–503.

Leon, M. (2002). Towards the individualization of social rights: Hidden familialistic practices in Spanish social policy. *South European Society and Politics*, *7*(3), 53–80.

Lewis, J., & Davies, C. (1991). Protective legislation in Britain, 1870–1990: Equality, difference and their implications for women. *Policy & Politics*, *19*(1), 13–25.

Lewis, J., & Giullari, S. (2005). The adult-worker model family, gender equality and care: The search for new policy principles and the possibilities and problems of a capabilities approach. *Economy and Society*, *34*(1), 76–104.

Manning, N. (2007). Turkey, the EU and social policy. *Social Policy & Society*, *6*(4), 491–501.

Michel, S. (2000). Introduction. *Social Politics, Special Issue: Beyond Maternalism*, *7*(1), 1–4.

Molyneux, M. (2007). *Change and continuity in social protection in Latin America: Mothers at the service of the state?* Gender and Development Programme Paper Number 1, United Nations Research Institute for Social Development.

Sainsbury, D. (1996). *Gender, equality, and welfare states*. Cambridge, NY: Cambridge University Press.

Savaşkan, O. (2007). *Contemporary social policy in Turkey: Workfare programs in the context of the neo-liberal international governance system*. M.A. thesis, Boğaziçi University.

SPF. (2007). *Boğaziçi Üniversitesi Sosyal Politika Forumu Bülteni*, 2. Retrieved from http://www.spf.boun.edu.tr/docs/SPFBulten-No2-Ocak07.pdf

SYDGM. (2008). *Şartlı nakit transferi – eğitim ve sağlık yardımları bilgi broşürü*. Retrieved from http://www.sydgm.gov.tr/Sydtf/Web/duyurular/SNTBROSUR2008SUBAT.doc

Toksöz, G. (2007). *Women's employment situation in Turkey*. Ankara: International Labor Office.

TÜİK. (2007). Retrieved from http://www.tuik.gov.tr

TÜSİAD. (2004). *Sağlıklı bir gelecek: Sağlık reformu yolunda uygulanabilir çözüm önerileri*. Istanbul: TÜSİAD.

UNDP. (2007). *Human development report 2007–2008*. New York: Palgrave Macmillan.

Üstündağ, N., & Yoltar, Ç. (2007). Türkiye'de sağlık sisteminin dönüşümü: bir devlet etnografisi. In Ç. Keyder & N. Üstündağ (Eds.), *Avrupa'da ve Türkiye'de sağlık politikaları* (pp. 55–93). Istanbul: İletişim.

World Bank. (2006). *Turkey: Labour market study*. Poverty Reduction and Economic Management Unit: Europe and Central Asia Region of the World Bank.

World Bank & SIS. (2005). *Joint poverty assessment report*. SIS & Human Development Sector Unit: Europe and Central Asia Region of the World Bank.

Yakut-Çakar, B., & Buğra, A. (2007). *Tackling child poverty in Turkey: A brief assessment of policies*. Independent Expert Report.

Yazıcı, B. (2007). *Social work and the politics of the family at the crossroads of welfare reform in Turkey*. Ph.D. dissertation, New York University.

Gender, Children and Families in the Greek Welfare State

Theano Kallinikaki

Introduction

Since the early 1990s there has been increased interest in the Greek welfare state and an attempt by social policy experts to categorize it within one of the main classification schemes offered by comparative social policy literature. Social policy experts have focused on the similarities the Greek welfare state shares with the other South European EU-member welfare states (Italy, Spain, and Portugal) and have concluded they constitute a discerning welfare structure (Ferrera, 1996; Petmesidou & Mossialos, 2006; Sotiropoulos, 2004; Matsaganis, 2002). The Greek welfare state is characterized as "corporatist" (Matsaganis, 2002), "continental" (Katrougalos, 1996), and as a "familist gender regime" (Davaki, 2006), with static, paternalistic, clientelist models of social organization (Petmesidou, 2006a). According to Lewis's (1992) classification of welfare regimes, the Greek welfare state is identified closest to the "strong male breadwinner cluster," which is characterized by low female participation in the labor market and full provision of care to children and the elderly by the female family members. As in other South European countries the welfare of Greek citizens of all ages depends on family arrangements and networks instead of on state provisions. This status quo reflects Flaquer's (2002) argument that "the welfare state in South Europe is the Mediterranean figure of family welfare."

Specific attention has been given to the particularities and the fragmented role of the Greek welfare state, which intervenes in selected cases, on behalf of individuals or groups, in an effort to maintain social peace and cohesion (Petmesidou, 2006b; Stasinopoulou, 2002). Emphasis is placed on public support of multi-children families (with at least four children, but since 2007 families with three are eligible for support as well) (Matsaganis, 2002; Mousourou, 2004). Social Policy researchers authors have documented the weakness and inefficiencies of the Greek welfare state in meeting its citizens' needs (Petmesidou, 2006b; Papatheodorou & Petmesidou,

T. Kallinikaki (✉)
Professor of Social Work, Department of Social Administration, Democritus University of Thrace, Komotini, Greece
e-mail: thkallin@socadm.duth.gr

M. Ajzenstadt, J. Gal (eds.), *Children, Gender and Families in Mediterranean Welfare States*, Children's Well-Being: Indicators and Research 2, DOI 10.1007/978-90-481-8842-0_9, © Springer Science+Business Media B.V. 2010

2006) while Taylor-Gooby has concluded that "it spends roughly the same as much of Europe, but is less effective in meeting the needs of its poorest citizens" (Taylor-Gooby, 2006).

Petmesidou's recent studies and comparative investigations offer a comprehensive description of the current development of the Greek and the South European welfare states, each within their own historical and social contexts. These studies have identified significant similarities and differences in social, economic, and political structures across Southern Europe by tracing the historical development in each area. In addition they have identified distinctive features including the lack of industrialization, a rapid change from an agrarian-based economy to a service-oriented economy, a large informal economy, the traditional contractual relations, a weak collective solidarity and civil society, the predominance of paternalistic, clientistic structures of the social organizations, and nonuniversal welfare provision except for a universal health system (Petmesidou, 2006a; Petmesidou & Mossialos, 2006; Papatheodorou & Petmesidou, 2006).

Despite the similarities between the Greek welfare state and other South European welfare states some significant differences must be taken into consideration. First of all, attempts to study the Greek welfare state must take into consideration the territorial structure of Greece, which is often overlooked in studies of other countries. The territorial aspect is particularly important as a result of the mainland–island and urban–rural divides in Greece. Both service development and service access is significantly different and complex for the inhabitants of island and rural areas. In addition, state and religion are not separated and religious affiliation in Greece is particularly strong. The Greek Orthodox Church is a powerful institution both politically and economically. It has an active involvement in the main political controversies and national issues, including the elimination of the notation of citizens' religious affiliation on identity cards, the practice of civil weddings and the legislation of gay and civil partnerships. In addition the Greek Orthodox Church influences educational and moral issues, policies and family values[1] and promotes negative perceptions of abortion and positive perceptions of traditional family roles and the family size (for example the provision of a generous benefit for the third child of Orthodox families in Thrace[2]). The Church provides its own means of social protection to the poorest parishioners in the form of donations of clothes and regular meals, and in the form of institutional care for elderly and unprotected children and adolescents. Last years its social provision was expanded to Greek citizens living abroad by the establishment of a nongovernmental organization (NGO).

Greek citizens, governments and social researchers have never been satisfied with the existing welfare model. In every day communication the term "welfare state" is synonymous with the provision of allowances to those who live in poverty, those

---

[1]One example (among many) is the official title of the "Ministry of Education and Religious Affairs."

[2]Thrace is located in northeast Greece, one of the most underdeveloped areas of Greece, where the only officially recognized minority (Muslims) resides.

who are neglected and permanently disabled and refers to social workers, the professionals who serve as the mediators in provision of these allowances. During the last 30 years the terms "welfare state expansion" and "reform" have become popular topics in the rhetoric of political parties and politicians, and of ministries and organizations. This rhetoric is a result of the interplay between domestic politics, changing family structures, and European influences, stemming from of the country's integration into the EU. Sectors of major importance, such as health and social care,[3] education, social security, and public administration are currently either undergoing reform or reform is planned for the future. Welfare reform must take into consideration new risks and social problems which emerge as a result of phenomenon including demographic ageing, continuing urbanization, changing gender roles, the increase in long-term (more than 1 year) and female unemployment, employment in the underground economy, and increased influx of immigrants.[4]

The aim of this chapter is to provide an outline of the changing structure and fluidity of the modern family and to summarize the main objectives of the reform in the sphere of family policy and other policies that affect families and children. The social work perspective of the author looks at the micro process taking place and takes into account a wide view of society's continuous change and recent evolution in the areas of employment and migration which affect families and children living in Greece.

Issues and problems faced by reform strategies will be dealt with in the first section of this chapter. The second section briefly reviews the emergence of gender issues as a concern of female employment policy. The third section presents changes that have taken place following developments in demographic ageing, urbanization, changing gender roles and employment patterns that have had a substantial impact on both family values and on family schemes. The fourth explores the formation of the welfare state with regard to the family and, in more detail, income support policies, including the absence of services supporting families and children. Finally, the fifth section focuses on mothers' employment reconciliation policies, and offers some recent data for processing.

---

[3]The most extensive reform was introduced by Law 2082/1992 on the "reorganization of social welfare and new methods of social welfare," which was replaced by Law 2646/1998 on the "Reorganization of the National System of Social Care and Other Provisions" which provided for the transition of the Centers for Family Care, from the state-run responsibility of the National Welfare Organization, to the second-tier local authorities in 2003 (1. 3106/03).

[4]Unquestionably, for Greece, which has traditionally been a country of emigration, the migrant waves produced serious, multifaceted economic and social effects. At the end of 2004 the number of immigrants was estimated to be 950,000 non-EU foreigners, mostly Albanians, Bulgarians, and Romanians, and 200,000 fellow Greeks (homogeneous). This is compared to the estimated total number of immigrants in 1991 which was 270,000 (Mediterranean Migration Observatory, 2005, p. 1). Immigrants are concentrated in the Municipality of Athens, some 132,000, 17% of total population, Thessaloniki, with 27,000 and 7% of local population, and some tourist islands close to the border with Albania. According to 2001 census data, immigrants, mostly illegal, consist of 10.3% of the Greek workforce and 7% of the total population. In 2007, 112,000 illegal immigrants entered the country.

Reform's Initiatives and Arrangements Affecting Families and Children

The high level of economic growth during the 1990s in Greece has not led to a considerable growth in employment, diminished poverty rates (the government did not introduce a guaranteed minimum income program for all groups at risk of poverty[5]), or a visible convergence among regions/prefectures (Petmesidou & Mossialos, 2006; Ministry of Economy, 2007). Social expenditure as a percentage of the Greek GDP has increased while the expenditure on social protection as a percentage of the GDP, grew from 21.2 in 1992 to 27.2 in 2001. When expenditure on social protection is measured in purchasing power standards (PPS) Greece lags behind most countries of the EU-15. In 2001 the PPS in Greece was 3.971 whereas the EU-15 average was 6.405.[6] Public expenditure on pensions has always been high; in fact in 2004 Greece paid the highest percentage (51.3%) in Europe (EU-15 average was 46%). Families and children were granted only 6.9% of the social budget and the unemployed received 6.0% as compared to the EU-15 which was 8.0 and 6.2%, respectively. After social transfer payments in Greece the percentage of persons at-risk of poverty fell from 23 to 20%, whereas the EU-27 average after transfers fell from 24 to 15% (European Commission, 2005). In 2007 the total expenditure for social protection dropped to 22.64% of GDP (Ministry of Employment and Social Security, 2007).

In the process of reforming policies concerning gender issues, the disabled, decentralization of services, employment, vocational training, regional development, policies of a high importance for families in different stages of their life cycle and children, Greece has adopted EU policy tools for consultation and decision making and implemented many programs, co-funded by the EU.

The Ioannis Kapodistrias Act, 2539/1997, was the most important reform. This institutional reform of the local administration merged 457 municipalities and 5,318 administrative communities across the country into 900 municipalities and 133 communities. Numerous state responsibilities were transferred to the municipalities (family advice centers, holiday camps for children, preschool and out-of-school care, and home care for the elderly) and local communities became able to participate in planning and implementing social and local development policies. Despite the inadequacies of these services as a result of funding and staff shortages and inexperience (Sotiropoulos, 2004; Kallinikaki, forthcoming), consumers overwhelmingly trust them because of their geographic and social proximity

---

[5]A measure for mature families is a means-tested, "social solidarity benefit" (EKAS), introduced in 1996, of 230€ (from 1/1/2008) that has been given to low income pensioners as a supplementary pension. Single people older than 65 without social insurance receive a monthly allowance of 266€ for housing assistance. In 2008 the Ministry of Economy established a National Fund for Social Cohesion "in order to reduce the risks of social exclusion aiming to define a new financial support for those at risk of poverty" (Ministry of Employment and Social Security, 2007).

[6]In 2001 the average social expenditure in the EU-15 was 27.5%, ranging from 14.6% in Ireland to 31.3% in Sweden, whereas Greece shared the eighth position with the UK (27.2%) (European Commission, 2005, pp. 42–43).

(as compared to the centralized public services) and support their permanent operation and further development (Stratigaki, 2004). Similarly, the establishment of Civil Service Offices in all second-tier local authorities was positively accepted by Greek citizens.

One important development was the establishment of various observatory bodies and specialized committees set up in order to collect, summarize, and document a wide range of "social" data. Although this data lacks any attention to the extent and depth of the social phenomenon under consideration and to the adopted policy processes and/or its effects, the purely numerical and statistical data does facilitate a basic study of these policies and social phenomenon.

The welfare reform included a number of programs co-funded by the EU and incorporated "good practices" for social integration in a wide range of areas and objectives. These had an impact on families and children of specific vulnerable groups of the population (i.e. the improvement of public accessibility for the disabled, the integrated action plan for Roma settlement 2002–2004, the settlement of those who were repatriated and school attendance policies for children of former inmates and immigrant children). In addition, significant efforts are being made to reduce adult illiteracy through adult education centers and second-chance schools. However, as a result of their pre-determined short duration and subsequent discontinuation, the lack of close interaction between them and of synergy with other crucial policies of economic growth and competitiveness, and their incompatibility with the procedures and the skills of the existing organizations and services these reforms were not sufficiently effective. Imitation programs promote "one size fits all" policies within Europe[7] which do not respond to the material or emotional needs of specific groups or to the culture of a local community, and do not adjust according to the living conditions of the recipients. For example, the participants in an allowance program for unemployed repatriated women refused to participate in personal counseling, stating: "we know how to raise our children, the thing that we need is a job and we need it now" (Zaimakis & Kallinikaki, 2004). Another example is the introduction of an annual benefit of 300€ for low income households (up to 3,000€ per year) with children between 6 and 16 years who are pupils of the 9-year-compulsory education, living in deprived, mountainous areas. As a result of the first implementation of this policy, a significant number of children who had not previously registered for school, or who had dropped out of school, registered. Unfortunately schools in these disadvantaged areas were uninformed of the policy and unprepared to welcome the significant wave of pupils due to lack of room and staff and the absence of an inclusive attitude towards them and their parents. Thus, the schools merely registered the students but did not actually teach them and thus the policy proved essentially ineffective.[8]

---

[7] As Ian Gough mentioned last April in his speech in Athens.

[8] Pupils living in these deprived areas, in mountainous areas or on the borders of the big cities, have the highest drop-out rate from compulsory education. These communities face severe socio-economic problems, high unemployment rates, and large numbers of illiterate adult population. People live in very poor housing, and in some cases there is not even running water and heating facilities. Interventions aiming to develop motives or incentives for the integration of these

Developments in legislation in fields such as decentralization of services for drugs addicts, foster care, and transfer of public services to the local authorities are significant, but have not been accompanied by essential reforms in service structures or by advanced staff training and new staff engagement. While some were introduced unilaterally, most of the new laws have to be interpreted by official decisions or documents signed by Ministers of the relevant Ministries. Some decisions were delayed for a long time due to related pending financial decisions, connected programs awaiting establishment, or the need to hire new professionals. Delays in construction, repair of buildings, or negative reactions by local residents because of the establishment of a social service close to their homes, produced further implementation delays or diminished their effects (from the outset, the allotted duration of the programs were shorter than needed for their effective establishment).

In the case of the National Health System the deficiency in primary care and the inefficient operation of the hospital care has significantly affected families. Thirty years after the establishment of the National Health System and despite the continuing efforts to improve its provisions, major geographical inequalities regarding the quality and infrastructure of medical care still persist. The development of primary medical and mental care in urban areas has been delayed, while both primary and secondary care in peripheral areas is limited. The private sector is particularly expanding in the maternity – gynecological, cardiac, and psychiatric fields.

The most recent reform of the social security system, which has had a significant effect on families and children, is focused on cutting the large number of social security organizations, increasing labor market participation, regulating pensions, and ensuring the long-term sustainability of the social security system especially in light of the rising financial needs as a result of demographic ageing, the health system and public finances. Although the reform of the social security system took place in the context of massive strikes and both worker and pensioner demonstrations, it did not include initiatives aimed at ensuring a "safety net" for all disadvantaged groups.

While many initiatives were aimed at reducing clientalism, this phenomenon has not been affected. Greek social welfare, and Greek society in general, is the victim of extensive clientalism. Clientalism affects all parts of Greek life; among other things it is a way of being trained, employed (mainly permanently), admitted for specific medical care, and accepted into a local community. As an integral part of the political and economic system, it hinders in-depth welfare reform and the adoption of universal, holistic policies for families and children.

---

children into primary schools and to encourage them to stay at school until they complete their 9-year compulsory education must be holistic (affecting aspects of individual, family, and social life that influence the relationship between children, their families, and school). For example, www.museduc.gr: *supporting minority pupils living in underdeveloped areas.*

Gender Issues

Gender is a relatively new issue in Greece, first introduced by the Greek women's movement in the early 1980s (after the restoration of democracy in 1974). The women's movement mainly contributed to legislative reform in favor of gender equality and women's self determination, which was defined for the first time by the new constitution, adopted in 1975. Gender-segregated schools were abolished and women entered the military service. Unsurprisingly the evolution of gender equality occurred during the socialist government (PASOK) as part of the 1983 family law and the legislation of other laws such as the "Implementation of Gender Equality in Employment Relations" (law 1414) and "Facility to Employees with Family Obligations" (law 1483).

Gender equalization policies in employment also occurred as a result of the Europeanization process in Greece, especially in areas where women were absent or less represented. Women entered the Merchant Marine Academies on equal terms as men without a quota. The direct result of this was an increased number of women in naval professions. In addition, since 2002 the ratification of the Code of the Hellenic Coast Guard (Law, 3079/2002) has abolished all quotas, which previously restricted women's access to the Coast Guard.

During the last decade a number of bodies were established in order to contribute, influence, and monitor the development and implementation of effective and inclusive policies and act against gender discrimination. The General Secretariat for Gender Equality, established by the Ministry of Interior, Public Administration, and Decentralization, is responsible for planning gender-equality policy in all fields. It supervises and finances the Center for Equality Issues (KETHI), an organization dealing solely with gender equality. In addition, it operates three advisory centers providing counseling and legal support services on matters of employment and entrepreneurship to women who belong to special categories, those threatened by social exclusion, those unemployed for a long-term period, and those over 45 years of age. Moreover, KETHI, as a coordinating agency, has implemented various projects promoting gender issues, which were co-financed by the European Commission (80%) and the General Secretariat for Gender Equality (20%). For example the project entitled "Equal Partners: Reconsidering men's role at work and private life," aimed at informing and raising public awareness, mainly of men and fathers, of the need to reconcile and harmonize their work obligations and family life by redefining stereotypes concerning the role of the father. In addition, in order to promote equality between women and men and combat stereotypes in the educational sphere, KETHI implemented the project "Training of Teachers and Intervention Programmes to Promote Gender Equality," which offered educational visits and informational lectures to teachers and pupils of the three last grades of elementary schools, secondary schools, and technical educational schools all over Greece.

The promotion of gender equality was also introduced in the tertiary education system at the graduate level (in eight universities and four technological educational institutes). These institutions aimed to reform their curricula and to include subjects on equality. Three universities offer postgraduate majors in equality issues and many others offer several research programmes on equality issues.

The Parliament passed law 3488/2006 in order to promote equal treatment of men and women in terms of access to employment and work relations, and the reduction of sexual harassment in the workplace. This law defined sexual harassment for the first time, tackling gender-based discrimination in the workplace, and created the legal stipulation to compensating victims. All forms of gender in terms of access to employment, and the establishment, evolution, and termination of employment in private and public sectors were also abolished.

Recently, a National Committee on Equality between men and women was established as a permanent social dialogue board (Art. 8 of the Law 3491/2006). The Committee's task is to contribute to the national strategy for equality between women and men, formulate necessary policies and measures and monitor their implementation, as well as evaluate their results both at the national and regional levels.

It must be noted that the EU policy of equality between women and men has been criticized. The EU policy is based on the idea of financial equality of women which comes from the liberal tradition. This tradition holds that women must integrate into the labor market by adopting required qualifications. This overlooks the existing structural gender inequality in areas with familial social structures, where discrimination of women is still reproduced (Scbunter-Kleemann, 2000).

Gender issues remain a priority for policy makers in Greece. The permissive "Administrative Reform 2007–2013" includes an axis entitled "reinforcing gender equality policy" aiming at "the improvement of quality and effectiveness of gender equality policies planned and implemented in the country, the integration of gender equality in the whole range of public action, at the level of central and local administration, and the reinforcement of the position and participation of women in the public and social sector, and, especially, in decision-making centers" (Ministry of Economy and Finance, 2007). The road to gender equality remains long. According to recent research undertaken by the Research Committee of Piraeus University (2008), women are paid 11% less than their male colleagues and they represent 9% of the members of Chambers, 7% of the members of the Board of Directors of the largest firms, and 15% of the existing enterprises are female.

Family and Family Policies in Greece

In Greece, marriage, maternity, and children are "under the protection of the state." This protection is officially defined by the Greek constitution (Article 21). This protection manifests itself mostly in the form of provision of financial aid to families, tax exemptions, allowances and subsidies, and less through the provision of services. Family policy does not exist as a distinct, autonomous field. It is promoted in pieces, through policies applied for personal rights, gender equality, and child-care rearing. Policies not specifically designed in relation to families, such as tax policies, social insurance and employment policies, impact families and women. Most ministries (Interior, Labor, Education, and Health) and state agencies make decisions that take into consideration domestic responsibilities, which usually include demographic implications. Although the role of the family as a welfare provider has been documented extensively by various studies, a systematic policy supportive of the multifarious needs of the families has not been developed. Family members gain access to delivered care only after they have been identified as members of a specific age and disadvantaged category group.

In Greece, as in the other Mediterranean countries, families are characterized by traditional roles and family solidarity is strong. The married, or remarried couple with children is the most common family structure. According to FFS in Greece the vast majority of people living with a partner are married (Symeonidou, 2002), and more than 90% of children in Greece live with both parents (UNICEF, 2007). Although the average number of persons per household has declined significantly, from 4.11 in 1951 to 2.80 in 2001, the majority of the population live in households of at least two persons (Symeonidou, 2002). The family unit is responsible for education, accommodation for the unmarried, care of offspring, and extra care in case of crisis (loss of employment, serious health problems). It traditionally served, and to an extent still continues to serve, as a "shock absorber" institution (Matsaganis & Tsakloglou, 2001, p. 192). Despite its increasing fluidity, family remains the most important provider of welfare and the mechanism of redistributing resources by filling in income gaps for first-time jobseekers and elderly family members (with low minimum benefits) and by providing childcare services.

As in other South European countries, in Greece the number of home owners is high (Castles & Ferrera, 1996), which is meant to diminish social insecurity both in the present and in the future. As Trifilletti (1998) has argued home ownership is a primitive form of security against social risks. It is encouraged by the loan policies for employees in the public sector and other categories of employees.

The most important change to the Greek family was introduced by the major reform of the Greek family law in 1983 (replacing the legislation dated from 1946). Following this reform, women are allowed to keep their surname after they get married and can have a legal residence different from that of their spouse. Furthermore, spouses now are able to make decisions together in regards to any marital issue and exercise parental care (the term "father's force" was abolished). The surname of children is determined by common declaration made before the wedding by both parents and can be the surname of either or both parents. Children born out of wedlock have equal rights to those born within marriage, except in regards to surname (that of the lone parent) and parental care. Important improvements include the introduction of divorce by mutual consent, the maintenance and claim to part of personal property of either spouse during marriage, the health insurance provision to divorced wives and widows through their ex-husbands, and the assignment of childcare to one of the two parents without any discrimination.

Since 1982 (Law 1250) the distinction between religious and civil marriage was created and the anachronistic institution of the dowry[9] was abolished. However, the tendency towards orthodox marriage remains strong and is supported by the Greek Orthodox Church.[10] More than 90% of marriages take place in Orthodox churches, and the remainder take place in municipalities (Eurostat, 2008).

Since 1986 abortion during the first 12 weeks after conception has been legal. Abortion can be performed after 12 weeks only in cases where there is a high risk to the health of either the embryo or the mother. This improvement was important because it permits the coverage of the medical procedure under social insurance and encourages young women to visit hospitals and gynecological clinics.

Demographic ageing and uncertain changing conditions in employment have affected family values and gender roles and have had a substantial impact on family structure. Fluidity, as a way of organizing private life, is the main characteristic of the modern Greek family (Mousourou, 2005). The occurrence of nontraditional family structures, especially that of the single parent family (10.9%, although it is the lowest in Europe), intercultural marriages, divorced parents and unmarried cohabitation (in 2001 it was 1%, but among the population between 16 and 29, the rate was 8%) have increased (Eurostat, 2004). These changes and the increase in births out of wedlock (1% in 1970 as compared to 4% in 2001) reflect an erosion of traditional family structures. Younger generations of both sexes are more likely to delay starting a family in favor of pursuing tertiary education. In 2006 the average age of a woman at the time of their first marriage was 28.2 years old, whereas in 1998 it was 25.9 years of age and in 1970 it was 22.9 years of age. Other demographic trends that have increased are the average age of women at the birth of their first child (29.8 in 2006 as opposed to 28.35 in 1996 and 26.2 in 1981), and the average life span (75.9 years for men and 81.0 for women in 2007 as opposed to 72.2 and 76.4 years respectively in 1981 and 67.3 years and 72.2 respectively in 1961) (Laboratory of Demographic and Social Analysis, 2007).

Marriage rates declined from 6.4 per 1,000 inhabitants in 1991, to 5.30 in 2001 and even further to 5.18 in 2006. The fertility rate dropped dramatically from 2.28 per 1,000 women in 1960 to 2.21 in 1980 and then to 1.29 in 2001 (Eurostat, 2004). The average duration of marriages has dropped and converged in the 1990s with the EU average of 12 years (Bagavos, 2002).

Divorce rates have increased from 96.9 per 1,000 inhabitants in 1981 to 101.2 in 2001 and then to 221.1 in 2005 (National Statistical Service of Greece, 2007). Marriage duration and number of children have a stabilizing effect on marriage; most of the dissolved marriages last at least 10 years (58%) and take place when

---

[9]Dowry was property given from a bride's parents to her husband as a precondition for marriage. It was considered as the basis for a good start of a daughter's married life. It has taken another form; that of immovable property given to children (daughters or sons) at the start of their independent life, usually when they get married.

[10]People who are married in a civil wedding are not allowed to baptize a baby (to be a godfather or a godmother) and cannot expect to have an orthodox funeral ceremony.

couples' children are between 7 and 18 years of age. Other factors related positively to the divorce rate are parental divorce of spouses, pre-marital cohabitation, religiosity, and place of origin. However, the employment and education of women are not related to divorce rates (Symeonidou, 2006). Moreover, the divorce rate was affected by the new legislation, which allowed for easier divorce processes. The quickest time needed for an official consent divorce is 12–18 months while the cost is at least 1,500€.

Changes have occurred in the way families live. Fathers of younger generations are more participatory in the responsibility for their children's care than in the past. The once strong tradition of daily shared family meals has recently changed and only 58.1% of parents report that they talk with their young children several times a week. This is lower than the average in OECD (Organization for Economic Cooperation and Development) countries (62.8%) (UNICEF, 2007).

As noted above, existing family policy is strained in terms of specific measures for those in serious need. Some are available for large families and those "at risk" or in a crisis situation. Extra tax regulations are made for families with disabled members and allowances are granted to the heavily disabled.[11]

The tax free income of 12,000€ increases by 1,000€ each for the first and second child, and increases to 6,000€ for the third child. Family and child allowances are given to all salaried employees (both spouses) in the public and private sector with children under 18 years of age or up to 21 if the children are students. A cash benefit of 2,000€ is provided to each mother after the birth of her third child. Parents with three or more children receive allowances (a monthly allowance for three or more children, a lifelong pension for the mother), and all family members are eligible for specific rights (reduced public transportation fares, reduced electricity and water supplement bills, tax release, duty free cars and housing). Children with two or more siblings receive priority places in kindergartens and in the employment force, they study in the universities that operate in or close to their family's place of residence, and the eldest son is drafted for 2/3 of the obligatory military training.

The clear preference for large families is evident from the universal provision that favors large families and from the fact that the allowances for these families are financed through the state budget; whereas marriage, maternity, and children allowances are dependant on employment and financed through employee contributions. Thus, unemployed spouses and parents are excluded from these provisions. Furthermore, due to the diversity of different insurance organizations, total provisions differ according to the employment sector, family income, and number of children (Matsaganis, 2002).

---

[11] Individuals with disability levels of 67% or more, unable to be employed are granted an allowance of 360€ per month. This allowance is administered by the welfare Ministry and financed by state off-budget, independent resources. For blind persons, the employed and pensioners receive 266€, students and lawyers 532€, whilst deaf people and those suffering from anemia receive 266€.

Policies supporting a family's structure include job-protected parental leave extended to fathers, paid leave, and flexible working hours. In addition, an employer cannot refuse to employ a woman on the grounds of pregnancy or recent childbirth, and a woman who has been on maternity leave can return to her work at an equivalent post, terms and conditions and can benefit from any improvement in work conditions. This protection also applies to working parents making use of parental leave to raise their children.

In the public sector maternity leave is guaranteed for 5 months (two before and three after birth) paid at 100% of existing salary, while in the private sector only 4 months is guaranteed. Mothers working in the public sector can choose between a 9-month breast-feeding paid leave or a reduced time schedule of either 2 h a day for 1 year following maternity leave or of 1 hour a day for 2 years. In the private sector mothers can work for 1 h less for 30 months after birth, or 2 h less for 12 months. Fathers can use this right when their wives do not use it. Unpaid parental leave (3.5 months for each parent in the private sector) and an additional maternity leave of 2 years for a child less than 6 years old, in the public sector, which increases by 1 year for each additional child, is available, but not generally used by working parents.

Single-mother households in Greece are more at risk of experiencing poverty and social exclusion (Kogidou, 1995). This group of single-mothers lives in low socio-economic conditions and lack resources and support, especially since in many cases the father has disappeared and they are thus more vulnerable to social exclusion and poverty. "Unprotected children" up to 16 years of age, living with their mother, receive a monthly allowance of 44€. Single parent families, like other family structures, in crisis situations (specifically "urgent socio-medical problems") are given an extra benefit of 234€ annually. Most of these households survive or have consumption patterns higher than their income due to informal support provided by the extended family (Bagavos, 2002).

Under the common EU policy perspective single mothers are considered among other vulnerable groups (persons with disabilities, former inmates, ex-drug addicts, immigrants) and can benefit from programs implemented for "employment and vocational training" and "new jobs and new self-employment entrepreneurships."[12]

The attitude within Greek society towards single parent families is seemingly contradictory. According to recent research[13] representatives of Greek social organizations, NGOs, and consumers of family policy measures argue that single mother households, those with many children, with disabled members, Roma families and

---

[12]Within the program "Employment and Vocational Training" specialized agencies provide social support services to the above-mentioned vulnerable population groups in order to develop their social and professional skills and facilitate their social inclusion.

[13]International research on "Improving Policy Responses and Outcomes to Socio-Economic Challenges" (IPROSEC) carried out during 2000–2003, in 11 countries, eight EU member states: France, Great Britain, Ireland, Greece, Italy, Spain, and Sweden and three under accession: Estonia, Hungary, and Poland.

families from other minority groups, require state provisions. On the other hand, the representatives of large families' associations have rejected measures supporting single parent families, claiming that they are responsible for the declining rate of nuclear families in the country (Stratigaki, 2004).

Services supporting familial relationships in the case of divorce or parent's temporary or persistent inability to fulfill their parental duties are limited, fragmented and according to research findings they are minimally accepted by citizens. NGO professionals stated that Greek adults believe that family issues must be solved independently within the family "because they are private issues and must be protected as such" (Stratigaki, 2004). The National Social Emergency Center which offers temporary accommodation, advice, and counseling in crisis situations, operates only in Athens and Thessaloniki and its service provision falls short of expectations set at the time of its establishment in 1998. A sort of gateway access to welfare services for families and children is through the Welfare Directorates of the prefectures situated in the capital of each prefecture, in addition to a number of the Centers for Family Care, recently transferred to the second-tier local authorities. These institutions provide very limited primary care services and family assistance as a result of staff shortages and the absence of an efficient link to other social and health services (Petmesidou, 2006b).

Because of a number of structural (service/professional shortages, provision of institutional childcare) and cultural reasons (grandparents replace automatically parents in crisis situations) foster care is underdeveloped in Greece (Kallinikaki, 2000). According to the National Organization of Social Care, the administrative office of the official state organization responsible for child protection, at the end of 2000 the total number of children in foster families was 596, while 1,277 children resided in residential care (Vergeti, forthcoming). However, the Greek Ombudsman (2006) reported in 2005 that the foster parent program was not put into operation. The introduction of "professional" foster care[14] did not impact its implementation except in some cases of relative foster care of long institutionalized mental health patients, which was introduced through the major reform of psychiatric care (Kallinikaki, 2000).

Adoption services are also not adequately developed and the adoption process is still slow and bureaucratic with long waiting lists of candidate adopters. Many of these candidate adopters turn to international social services or adoption services (mostly to Balkan or Asian countries). According to the national register of adoptions during 2005, 603 adoptions were carried out in Greece. These were 322 boys and 281 girls, and more than half (324) of the adoptees were born into marriage (Institute of Social Protection and Solidarity, 2007).

---

[14]The cash monthly benefit is 260€ per child, 340€ when the child or adult is disabled, 450€ in case of severe disabilities, and 850€ when the child is HIV-positive.

Children

When we discuss children's welfare or social needs in Greece, we refer to 1,660,899 under the age of 15, who constitute about 15.5% of the total resident population (10,934,097, 2001-Census),[15] and to the approximately 150,000 immigrant children under 15, mostly from Albania, other Balkan countries and Poland, who live in the country.

The Greek family is child-oriented and parents invest in their children's future living conditions and specifically in their earning potential through investment in education. Article 16 of the Greek constitution defines all levels of education in public institutions as free for all Greek citizens. Parents are legally obliged to send their children to school for a minimum of 9 years. Required school books for all subjects and at all levels of education are provided for free to all students. Furthermore, transportation to mandatory education is provided free of charge to students who live far from schools. It is also noteworthy that foreign minors living in Greece both legally and illegally are obligated to the same minimum school attendance as the native minors. Recently, the government, aiming to enable access to the educational institutions, introduced two new annual, financial contributions. Families with children studying in universities in cities other than the place of their residence are now eligible for 1,000€ assistance per academic year (Law 3220/2004) and families, whose annual income is no more than 3,000€ and have children up to 16 years of age who attend public schools are eligible for 300€ per school year. Law 3518/2006 revised the admission conditions for preschool education; children can begin attending kindergarten after they turn four and are obligated to attend kindergarten after they turn five.

Public education is free of charge and since the academic year of 2008–2009 included two foreign languages. At least one of these languages is usually English. However, parents of secondary school students, especially during the second half of secondary school, pay a significant amount in order to support their children's achievement and to prepare them for national examinations required for university studies.[16] In addition, families supplement their children's education with private tutorials, foreign languages, music, and athletics. Parents supplement their income with small-scale entrepreneurial activity or occasional, unstructured contracts with the labor market (i.e. seasonal work, day-laborers, working from home). Increased unemployment among university graduates has not diminished the new generations' positive orientation towards university studies. However, they tend to select subjects appointed to a qualified profession or those related to a position in the labor market.

Unquestionable developments have occurred in the education of disabled children. Disabled persons now have free access to universities without examinations.

---

[15]This is below the average percentage of children per total resident population in the European Union.

[16]The Ministry of Education introduced "additional instruction" and "complementary training" measures offered in the schools as after-school classes in order to reduce the private lessons' rate but this did not affect the attitudes of students and parents, who trust them more.

Law 2817/2000 encourages the integration of disabled pupils into general schools by providing them with tutorial classes but it also continues to allow divided education outside the framework of general education. Special units operate for children between 4 and 14 years of age, another for those between 14 and 18 and general and technical units for those between 18 and 22. The operation of "reception classes"[17] and tutorial classes for disabled pupils, in general schools, did not attract all of them. During the 2003–2004 school year 4,355 disabled pupils studied in 209 special school units of all levels (between 4 and 22 years of age) (NSSG, 2008).

Although corporal punishment in schools and general violence against children has been prohibited by law since 1998, there are parents and teachers who use physical punishment as a disciplinary method. In the last two decades cases of violence against children have surfaced and television panels and news programs have engaged in long discussions on the subject. While a number of child-abuse cases are reported to the Children Rights Department and various NGOs, additional cases remain hidden. In comparison to other OECD countries, Greek minors experience more violence in the form of physical fighting and less violence in the form of bullying (UNICEF, 2007).

With regard to prevention and regulation of domestic violence, a new law 3500/2006 prohibits domestic violence, perpetrated by all family members independent of their age. In addition, the law defines the punishment for "interfamily corporal damage" in accordance with its severity and the ability of the victim to resist. Victims are entitled to supportive social services and teachers who observe any violent mark on a pupil's body are required to report it to the District Attorney or to the nearest police station.

Greece has enacted laws, ratified international conventions, and adopted a number of measures all in order to promote and advance children's rights. The National Observatory of the Rights of Children, the Ombudsman' Department of Child's Rights[18], and the Child Health Institute are among the institutions dealing specifically with children's rights. Since 1989, the minimum employment age in the labor force, family businesses, agricultural, forestry, fishing and livestock sectors, has been 15. Adults who force minors under their care to beg for financial benefit are sentenced to a term in prison.

Since 1973, the state-run orphanages have been converted into childcare centers and the schools that previously operated inside them were closed or converted into

---

[17] Reception classes are those that welcome foreign pupils or pupils who have delayed starting school aiming to improve their social and communicative skills (language etc.) and to prepare for their participation in the general classes.

[18] The Children Rights Department during its 4.5 years of operation (until 13.12.2007) accepted 1,108 references. 38.1% of those references related to violations of children's rights in educational issues – mostly issues concerning organization and delivery of supportive measures for weak pupils and their school access. However, 18.7% of the cases related to family and childcare substitutes. A significant number of references related to the welcome conditions and health–social care issues of immigrant and refugee minors. (http:/www.synigoros.gr/0-18/gr/children and http:/www.e-paideia.et).

general schools. Since 1960 a benefit has been given to "unprotected children," under the age of 14, who are defined as orphans (those who have lost either parents or just their father), children whose fathers cannot support them because of health reasons, drug addiction or prison, and children born out of wedlock. This benefit was 44€ in December 2008. Children who live in childcare centers or in institutions do not qualify for this allowance.

Minors, both those with and without special needs, under the age of 18, who experience abuse, neglect, or live conditions which risk their well-being (physical or mental) can be placed either in foster families or in the very limited hostels located in the capital cities. Most of them live in anachronistic institutions, which remain the main solution. SOS Child Villages have been expanding in parallel with residential care offered by NGOs. The residential care for abused and neglected children and for chronically ill and severely disabled children has eluded the attention of the social care reform. Moreover, health insurance schemes do not include long-term domiciliary social care in rehabilitation centers or in homes for the chronically ill.

Parents, Usually Mothers – Employment Reconciliation

Employment in Greece has four major characteristics: extensive self employment (32% in 2001), low levels of part-time employment (4% of total employment), very low levels of part-time work (the lowest among EU countries), and extensive informal employment (private practice of disciplines, teaching foreign language lessons, working from home). Traditionally men were employed full-time while women were employed part-time in small family businesses and agriculture. During the period of socialist government in the 1980s the public sector expanded significantly. Because of the stability, permanent character, reliable salary payment and allowances of the public sector, employment in this sector is preferred over the unstable, short-term contracts and conditions linked to productivity that characterize the private sector.

Recently there has been a significant reduction of employment in industry and agriculture. While in 1990 27% of those employed worked in industry, in 2001 only 24% were employed in this field. In agriculture the percentage employed has reduced from 23% in 1990 to 16% in 2001. Simultaneously a rapid expansion of employment in the service sector has occurred from 50% in 1990 to 60% in 2001 (European Commission, 2002). Employment rates, especially of women, are still low. In 2001, the women who were employed, or were actively seeking work, constituted approximately 49% of women of working age whereas the EU-15 average was 60% (European Commission, 2002).

According to Korpi (2000), welfare state support for dual income families must be assessed according to three indicators: the public day care services for children between 0 and 2 years of age, paid maternity and paternity leave, and public home assistance for the elderly. These three indicators are in a transitional stage in Greece. Care services, both for children and the elderly, operated by local authorities, municipalities, and the ministry of education have recently increased and since 2001 many public primary schools adopted an extended timetable (ending at 4 p.m.).

Admission eligibility for preschool education was revised in 2006 (Law 3518/2006), as was described in the section about children above, and includes two possible years of education with a mandatory second year (for children that are 5 years old). In the case of children with special needs, the situation is more complex. The majority of these students are taught in state special schools that follow the official calendar of the mandatory schools (starting day, free days, holidays) but are not full-day schools, instead finishing at 1 p.m.

Despite the considerable development of the private sector in provision of care, many employed women depend on elderly relatives for childcare, while many others pay a significant portion of their salary to immigrant women for childcare. In Greece 14% of women between 45 and 49 years old live in cohabitation with three or more generations. This high rate of cohabitation among the generations indicates the important role played by women as caretakers for their grandchildren while parents work outside the home. This trend serves to substitute the weak and inefficient welfare state (Symeonidou, 2002). According to FFS findings (2004) 46.4% of the childcare for children under 3 years old with two working parents is the responsibility of grandparents.

Municipalities and communities throughout Greece have welcomed the program "Help at Home" (in 1998) for persons over 65 years of age and for the disabled, who live alone. However, this program is not subsidized for people who need continuous care (Amera, Stournara, & Manara, 2002). Most of the people in long-term, continued care are cared for by their daughters, daughters-in-law,[19] or by 24-h immigrant nurses (Triantafillou & Mestheneos, 2001). Private-sector institutional care for the elderly is rapidly increasing in urban areas. However, admission into these institutions is not a socially accepted solution to elderly caretaking. Less than 1% of those 65 years and older reside in an institution in both for-profit and the not-for-profit sectors. This is lower than the EU average (8–11%) and lower then the average in other South European countries (3% in Italy) (Ackers & Dwyer, 2002).

In 2006, the total employment rate was 61%. Female employment stood at 47.4%, while male employment was 74.6%. In 2006 the rate of the population between 15 and 64 years of age was 67.0%; that of women was 55.0% and that of men was 79.1%. Employment rates of women in Greece are lower than that in other Southern European countries and in the EU at large. In addition, employment rates of young women depend on whether they have children or not, with the rates dropping among women with children (Table 1). The employment rate of older workers (aged 55–64) was 42.3% in 2006. 26.6% of women in this age group were employed, which was significantly lower than the corresponding rate of men (59.2%).

---

[19] A payment or allowance for this hard job has been demanded by interested associations since the middle of the 1980s, but remains unfulfilled (Triantafillou & Mestheneos, 2001).

Table 1 Employment rates of women and men (aged 25–49), depending on whether they have children (under 12) – 2006

	Without children		With children		Difference	
	Women	Men	Women	Men	Women	Men
EU 27	76.0	80.8	62.4	91.4	−13.6	10.6
Greece	64.1	82.5	57.0	96.8	−7.0	14.3
Italy	66.7	80.7	54.6	93.8	−12.1	13.1
Portugal	77.3	82.7	76.4	94.2	−0.9	11.5
Spain	75.5	84.3	58.8	93.2	−16.7	8.8

Source: Extracted from Eurostat, European Labour Force Survey, annual averages (European Commission, 2008)

Table 2 Long-term unemployment rate – females

	1995	2000	2003	2006
EU (27)	–	4.6	4.5	4.0
EU (15)	5.8	4.1	3.7	3.5
Greece	8.1	10.1	8.9	8.0
Italy	10.0	8.4	6.6	4.5
Portugal	3.2	2.0	2.7	4.4
Spain	16.4	7.4	7.7	2.8

Source: Extracted from http://epp.eurostat.ec.europa.eu/portal/page

According to the latest available data of the National Statistical Service the downward trend of unemployment continued in 2007. In fact, women's unemployment rate dropped to 12.6% according to data of the 2nd quarter of 2007 (NSSG, 2007) but the long-term unemployment rate has remained stable for the last 10 years (Table 2). The structure of unemployment per age group shows increased rates of unemployment among young people between 15 and 24 years of age. The unemployment rate of young people in 2006 was 25.2%. However, the fact that the National Statistic Service does not consider those who participate in short-term job training, stage positions (of 4 months), or seasonal jobs as unemployed, must be taken into consideration.

According to data provided by the Greek Manpower Employment Organization (OAED)[20] in 2007 there were 434,996 unemployed people and 328,654 people

---

[20]Under the Ministry of Labor and Social Security, OAED operates decentralized offices which provide regular information on the availability of different categories of unemployed persons and on the incentives offered for their employment. It also provides activities to strengthen the position of the unemployed and develop the conditions for matching labor supply and demand (counseling on job seeking, training in utilizing specific tools like drafting a curriculum vitae and improving interview skills, etc). 625,000 people benefited from employment programmes such as "New Jobs", "New Self-Employed Programme" and "Stage", from 1/1/2006 to 30/4/2007 (Ministry of Employment and Social Security, 2007).

seeking employment. The unemployment benefit is 440€ per month for 12 months after the end of a job contract and is among the lowest in the EU-15 especially for unemployed single people and unemployed married couples. The unemployment benefit for a couple with two children replaces 44% of the previous earnings (the EU-15 average is 70%), for a single unemployed person the benefit replaces 41% of pervious earnings and for a single parent with two children the benefit replaces 47% of the previous earnings. Relative to other EU countries, unemployment support is lower when a number of different factors are taken into account. First of all, average wages in Greece are among the lowest in Europe. In addition no safety net exists for the unemployed after the entitlement to the insurance benefit has expired and finally, the monetary value of the benefit package for the unemployed continually erodes (Papadopoulos, 2006).

Women's participation in the work force has recently been promoted through increased incentives for "feminine entrepreneurship". OAED has undertaken a project allowing women who have children under 6 years old, or who take care of relatives with disabilities, to use their own residence as the headquarters of their enterprise. Moreover, the above-mentioned equality bodies (General Secretariat for Gender Equality) have initiated the project "Positive Actions in Favor of Women in Small, Medium, and Large Enterprises" which assists women working in these kinds of enterprises to obtain additional qualifications in order to promote their career on more favorable terms. Furthermore, the Research Center for Gender Equality has implemented a programme providing counseling services to women from disadvantaged groups who participate in the labor market. These services are aimed at encouraging women to enter the labor market, supporting their entrepreneurial activities, and promoting continued employment of women.

Concluding Remarks

As a result of the partial and deficient development of the Greek welfare state, the contemporary focus on "vulnerable groups" has effectively reproduced existing power relations and preserved the disempowering approaches intended to prevent absolute misery. Welfare arrangements suffer from serious imbalances and instability, which in turn cause inequalities, inefficiencies, and the lack of initiatives aimed at tackling paternalistic, clientelistic structures of the social organizations. Moreover, these arrangements do not promote the prevention and deinstitutionalization of the chronically ill – disabled infants, children, and adolescents.

The increased fluidity of the modern family, which is characterized by growing rates of nuclear and single-parent families and increased female participation in the labor force, limits its capacity to "protect" fellow family members in need. However, the family unit remains the most important provider of welfare and mechanism for the redistribution of resources.

Policies impacting the family unit are fragmented and are more demographically focused. The allocation of resources for children and the elderly have been introduced in order to encourage female participation in the labor market and support the reconciliation of domestic and professional responsibilities, and thus are aimed at reducing the domestic care responsibilities of women. Moreover, these policies do not take into consideration any pedagogical and psycho-social aspect of child development; for example the long-term impact of a reduced bond between mother and child.

The Greek family is child-oriented whereas Greek social policy emphasizes allowances and services that are client-oriented. Any reform responding to the weakness of the Greek welfare state discussed in this paper must undoubtedly focus on the implementation of a cohesive family policy and the development of family community services aimed at providing pluralistic and holistic approaches to native, immigrant and refugee families and children.

Despite shortcomings, improvements have taken place and the specific needs of excluded populations have been increasingly fulfilled. Limited attention is given to personal and social rights, refugees and asylum seekers are not adequately protected.

Reforming a residual, undeveloped, familialist, clientalist regime, like Greece, is not an easy, quick process. Furthermore, this process was not a national/subnational demand initiated by citizens associations, local communities, or by the organizations themselves, nor was there a consensus with regard to how the needs of the general population and specific groups could be facilitated.

Future improvements are expected to support regional initiatives to promote a strategic approach to social care, anti-poverty initiatives and to contribute to preventive, not merely curative, requirements.

References

Ackers, L., & Dwyer, P. (2002). *Senior citizenship – Retirement and welfare in the European Union*. Bristol: The Policy Press.

Amera, A., Stournara, A., & Manara, A. (2002). *Program help at home: Implementation report*. Athens: Central Union of Municipalities and Communities (Greek).

Bagavos, C. (2002). *General monitoring report on the situation of families in Greece*. Vienna: European Observatory on the Social Situation, Demography and Family – Austrian Institute for Family Matters.

Baldwin-Edwards, M. (2005). *Statistical data on immigrants in Greece: An analytic study of available data and recommendations for conformity with European Union standards*. Athens: Mediterranean Migration Observatory.

Castles, F. G., & Ferrera, M. (1996). Home ownership and the welfare state: Is Southern Europe different. *South European Society and Politics, 1*(2), 163–184.

Davaki, K. (2006). Family policies from a gender perspective. In M. Petmesidou & E. Mossialos (Eds.), *Social policy developments in Greece* (pp. 263–285). London: Ashgate.

European Commission. (2002). *Employment in Europe*. Luxembourg: Office of Official Publications of the European Communities.

European Commission. (2005). *The social conditions in European Union 2004*. Luxembourg: Office of Official Publications of the European Communities.

European Commission. (2008). *Report on Equality between women and men 2008*. Luxembourg: European Communities.

Eurostat. (2004). *European social statistics: Social protection expenditure and receipts.* Luxembourg: European Communities.

Eurostat. (2008). *European social statistic: Social protection expenditure and receipts.* Retrieved from http://epp.eurostat.ec.europa.eu/portal/page

Ferrera, M. (1996). The "Southern model" of welfare social Europe. *Journal of European Social Policy, 6*(1), 17–37.

Flaquer, L. (2002). Is there a special model of family policy in Southern Europe? In L. Maratou-Alipranti (Ed.), *Families and welfare state in Europe: Trends and challenges in the twenty-first century* (pp. 47–84). Athens: Gutenberg (Greek).

Greek Ombudsman. (2006). *Annual Report 2005.* Retrieved from http:/ www.synigoros.gr/annual _2005_ gr.htm

Institute of Social Protection and Solidarity. (2007). *Report 2005–2006.* Athens: Institute of Social Protection and Solidarity (Greek).

Kallinikaki, T. (2000). Foster care for mentally ill adults in Greece. In National Organization of Social Care (Ed.), *Foster care* (pp. 207–218). Athens: Greek Letters (Greek).

Kallinikaki, T. (2010, forthcoming). *Tracking the rights of prevention and primary intervention in the health, mental health and welfare systems.* In National Observatory for Children Rights (Ed.), The child rights in Greece of 21st century. Athens: Nea Genia (Greek).

Katrougalos, G. (1996). The South European welfare model: The Greek welfare state in search of an identity. *Journal of South European Social Policy, 6*(1), 39–60.

Kogidou, D. (1995). *Single-parent families: Reality, prospect, social policy.* Athens: Nea Synora (Greek).

Korpi, W. (2000). Faces of inequality: Gender, class and patterns of inequalities in different types of welfare states. *Social Politics, 7*(2), 27–191.

Laboratory of Demographic and Social Analysis. (2007). *Demographic profile of Greece 2007.* Volos: University of Thessaly (Greek).

Lewis, J. (1992). Gender and the development of the welfare regime. *Journal of European Social Policy, 2*(3), 159–173.

Matsaganis, M. (2002). Social policy and family in Greece. In L. Maratou-Alipranti (Ed.) *Families and welfare state in Europe: Trends and challenges in the twenty-first century.* (pp. 161–186). Athens: Gutenberg (Greek).

Matsaganis, M., & Tsakloglou, P. (2001). Social exclusion and social policy in Greece. In D. G. Mayers, J. Bergman, & R. Salais (Eds.), *Social exclusion in European social policy.* (pp. 188–203). Cheltenham: Edward Elgar.

Ministry of Economy and Finance. (2007). *National reform program 2005–2008: Implementation report 2007.* Athens: Ministry of Economy and Finance.

Ministry of Employment and Social Security. (2007). *Social budget 2007.* Athens: General Secretariat of Social Security.

Mousourou, L. (2004). Employment: and family life. In L. Mousourou & M. Stratigaki (Eds.), *Social policy issues* (pp. 73–106). Athens: Gutenberg (Greek).

Mousourou, L. (2005). *Family and family policy.* Athens: Gutenberg.

National Statistical Services of Greece (NSSG). (2007). *Greece in figures.* Athens: NSSG.

Papadopoulos, Th. (2006). Support for the unemployed in a Familistic Welfare Regime. In M. Petmesidou & E. Mossialos (Eds.), *Social policy developments in Greece* (pp. 219–238). London: Ashgate.

Papatheodorou, C., & Petmesidou, M. (2006). Poverty profiles and trends. How do southern European countries compare with each other? In M. Petmesidou & C. Papatheodorou (Eds.), *Poverty and social deprivation in the Mediterranean: Trends, policies and welfare prospects in the new millennium* (pp. 47–94). London: Zed Books.

Petmesidou, M. (2006a). Tracking social protection: Origins, path peculiarity, impasses and prospects. In M. Petmesidou & E. Mossialos (Eds.), *Social policy developments in Greece* (pp. 25–54). London: Ashgate.

Petmesidou, M. (2006b). Social care services: Amidst high fragmentation and poor initiatives for change. In M. Petmesidou & E. Mossialos (Eds.), *Social policy developments in Greece* (pp. 319–358). London: Ashgate.

Petmesidou, M., & Mossialos, E. (2006). Addressing social protection and policy in Greece. In M. Petmesidou & E. Mossialos (Eds.), *Social policy developments in Greece* (pp. 1–21). London: Ashgate.

Scbunter-Kleemann, S. (2000, May). *Gender mainstreaming as a strategy for modernising gender relations*. European Commission: European Observatory on Family Matters.

Sotiropoulos, D. A. (2004). The EU's impact on the Greek welfare state. Europeanization on paper. *Journal of European Social Policy*, *14*(3), 267–284.

Stasinopoulou, O. (2002). *Modern Social Policy Issues. From the Welfare State to "new" welfare pluralism. Care and aging – the modern pluralistic challenge*. Athens: Gutenberg.

Stratigaki, M. (2004). State interventions in the private life of the family. Prospects of the family policy. In L. Mousourou & M. Stratigaki (Eds.), *Social policy issues* (pp. 293–328). Athens: Gutenberg (Greek).

Symeonidou, H. (2002). *Fertility and family surveys in countries of ECE region: Standard country report – Greece*. New York and Geneva: United Nations.

Symeonidou, H. (2006). *Divorce Greece: country report*. Retrieved from www.iue.it/personal/Dronkers/divorce/Symeonidou.pdf

Taylor-Gooby, P. (2006). Greek welfare reform in a European context. In M. Petmesidou & E. Mossialos (Eds.), *Social policy developments in Greece* (pp. 405–411). London: Ashgate.

Triantafillou, J., & Mestheneos, E. (2001).Greece. In I. Philip (Ed.), *Family care of older people in Europe* (pp. 75–95). Amsterdam: IOS Press.

Trifilletti, R. (1998). Restructuring social care in Italy. In J. Lewis (Ed.), *Center social care and welfare state restructuring in Europe* (pp. 175–206). Aldershot: Ashgate.

UNICEF. (2007). *Child poverty in perspective: An overview of child well-being in rich countries, Innocenti Report Card 7*. Florence: Innocenti Research Centre.

Vergeti, A. (2009). *Clinical social work with families in crisis situations*. Athens: Topos (Greek).

Zaimakis, G., & Kallinikaki, T. (2004). *Locality and multiculturalism. Sapes Thrace*. Athens: Greek Letters (Greek).

Part IV
A Cross-National Comparison

Is There a "Mediterranean Welfare State"? A Country-Level Analysis

Anat Guy

Introduction

In the context of examining the Mediterranean welfare states, this chapter carries out a country-level analysis in order to uncover the common characteristics, as well as the differences, between the eight countries in this region. The chapter is divided into three sections: the first section draws a portrait of the demographic characteristics of the eight countries, the second section contains key aspects of social life in those countries, and the third section introduces key data concerning social aspects of the welfare state. This third and final section attempts to link the demographic characteristics and aspects of social life of each country to the respective welfare state. This contribution is analyzed in a comparative perspective.

The data presented in this chapter was taken from a variety of sources including: UNECE, UNdata, WHO, ISSA, the European Commission, Corruption Perceptions Index, OECD, the World Value Survey, CIA, and the central bureau of statistics of the different countries.

Demographic Aspects

Table 1 indicates major demographic differences between the eight Mediterranean countries.

Turkey has the largest population (73.1 million) of the eight, followed by Italy (53 million) and Spain (43 million). The two smallest countries are Cyprus and Malta, both with a population of under a million people (0.8 and 0.4, respectively). The other countries – Portugal, Israel, and Greece – each have populations of around 10 million. In all of the eight countries, the life expectancy for women is higher than that of men. However, the life expectancy for both men (69.1) and women (74) in

A. Guy (✉)
Department of Behavioral Sciences, College of Management Academic Studies,
Hebrew University, Rishon LeZion, 75190 Jerusalem, Israel
e-mail: msgai@mscc.huji.ac.il

M. Ajzenstadt, J. Gal (eds.), *Children, Gender and Families in Mediterranean Welfare States*, Children's Well-Being: Indicators and Research 2,
DOI 10.1007/978-90-481-8842-0_10, © Springer Science+Business Media B.V. 2010

Table 1 Demographic data

	Total population (millions)	Life expectancy at birth: total	Life expectancy at birth: men	Life expectancy at birth: women	Total fertility rate	Average annual rate of population change for 2005–2010, medium variant	Main Religion
Cyprus	0.8	78.15	76.7	n.a	1.6	1.06	Greek Orthodox
Greece	11.1	79.3	77.2	81.9	1.3	0.21	Greek Orthodox
Israel	7.11	80.61	78.8	82.5	2.8	1.66	Judaism
Italy	58	80.4	78.6	84.1	1.4	0.13	Roman Catholicism
Malta	0.4	79.8	77	81.9	1.4	0.43	Roman Catholicism
Portugal	10.5	78.2	75.5	82.3	1.5	0.37	Roman Catholicism
Spain	43	80.7	77.7	84.4	1.4	0.77	Roman Catholicism
Turkey	73.1	71.4	69.1	74	2.2	1.26	Islam
OECD average		78.6	75.7	81.1	1.6		

Average annual rate of population change for 2000–2005, medium variant % religious person – United Nations World Population Prospects: 2006 revision – Table A.8.

World Value Survey.

Data on OECD from OECD.Stat.

Sources: Life expectancy at birth, women (2006) UNECE; Life expectancy at birth, men (2006) UNECE; Total fertility rate (2006) UNdata; Cyprus WHO

Turkey is much lower in comparison to the other seven countries (women – 81.6–84.4; men – 76.7–78.8). Another point of interest is the range of fertility rates in the different countries: while in Cyprus, Greece, Italy, Malta, Portugal, and Spain fertility rates range from 1.3 to 1.6, they are significantly higher in Israel (2.8) and Turkey (2.2). These two countries (Israel and Turkey) are the only non-EU countries as well as the only non-Christian countries (majorities of Jews and Muslim, respectively) included in this review. Turkey and Israel also have the highest average percentage of annual growth. Another area that distinguishes between the six EU, predominantly Christian countries and the two non-EU and non-Christian countries is population structure, as illustrated in Graph 1 .

Turkey and Israel are "young countries" with a high percentage of young children under the age of 14 (37.14 and 28.35, respectively), and comparatively small percentages of elderly residents over the age of 65 (4.21 and 9.91, respectively). Nevertheless, it is important to note that in all eight countries the percentage of the population between the ages 15–64 range between 58.65 (Turkey) and 69.7 (Malta). This data shows that although almost two-thirds of the population in these countries is neither young nor old, their population composition is still different. The populations of Turkey and Israel both have a large percentage of young children and a relatively small percentage of elderly people, while the rest of the countries share a larger percentage of elderly people and a smaller or equal percentage of young children.

■ % of population aged 0-14 years   ■ % of population aged 15-64 years

■ % of population aged 65+ years

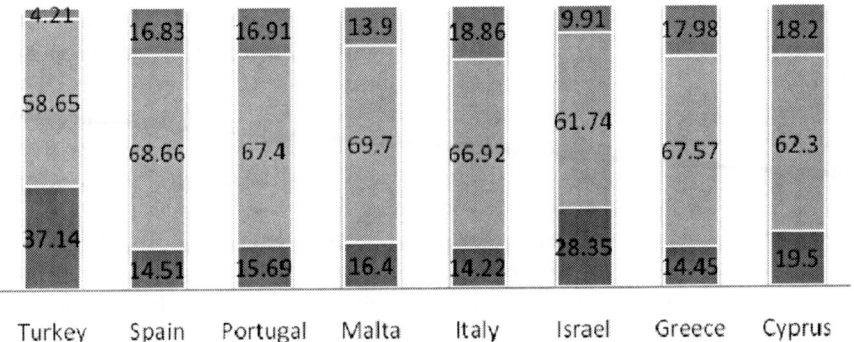

Graph 1 Population structure

From the demographic data one can conclude that while the eight Mediterranean countries differ in population size, the predominantly Christian countries (Cyprus, Greece, Italy, Malta, Portugal, and Spain) share demographic characteristics such as fertility rate, average annual percentage of growth and age demographics. Turkey and Israel, both non-Christian countries, share similar age demographics and fertility rates. It would appear, as has been claimed (Lindh, 1999; Lindh & Malmberg, 1999) that the high fertility rates in these countries affect the age demographics in these countries. In other words, high fertility rates result in a "younger society" with a higher percentage of young children in the country, while low fertility rates result in an "older society" in which the percentage of young children is equal or lower than the percentage of older people.

Social Aspects

The levels of wealth, inequality, and employment in each country are examined in Table 2.

The two wealthiest countries included in this study are Italy and Spain, both with income inequality (GINI) levels similar to the OECD average. Cyprus and Greece share similar GDP levels but differ in income inequality (GINI): while Cyprus has lower income inequality in comparison to the OECD average, Greece has a slightly higher income inequality than the average in the OECD. Israel, Portugal, and Malta have similar GDP per capita levels, but while Malta has the lowest level of income inequality among the eight countries, Israel and Spain have significantly high levels of income inequality, second only to Turkey, the poorest country with the highest income inequality.

Data on employment reflects a different aspect of wealth and inequality. Cyprus has the highest rate of employment as well as the lowest rate of unemployment. The data on unemployment rates indicates that most of these countries range between 6.1 and 8.5% of unemployment. Turkey has the highest unemployment rate at 8.5%.

According to Table 2, it is possible to distinguish between the eight countries and to divide them into three groups: Cyprus, Portugal, and Spain with a high percentage of total population participating in the labor force (71–69%, respectively); Israel, Italy, Malta, and Greece with slightly lower percentages of total population participating in the labor force (62–67%, respectively); and Turkey with the lowest percentage of total population participating in the labor force (55%). Unemployment data reveals, again, three groups of countries: Cyprus, with a very low unemployment rate (3.9%); Italy, Malta, and Israel with medium unemployment rates (6.1–7.3%), and the other countries with higher unemployment rates (8.1–8.5%).

The other indicators, including total employment growth rate and the average annual growth in the percentage of woman employed, show that there is no apparent connection between the two indicators. In Spain, for example, the total employment growth rate is very modest, only 1.1%, while the average annual growth in percentage of woman employed is high (4.23%) as compared to other countries.

The data shown in Table 3 reflects some additional aspects of social life in the eight countries examined.

The data refers to the corruption perception index (CPI), which implies the level of corruption (frequency and/or size of bribes) in the public and political sectors of each country, using data from 13 sources from 11 independent institutions

Table 2 Wealth and inequality

	GDP per capita (USD)	Income inequality (GINI)	Unemployment Rate (2007)	Employment rate	Labor force (% of total population ages 15–64)	Total employment growth rate (2007)	Employment rates: women (Average annual growth in percentage)
Cyprus	27,047	0.29	3.9	68.7	71	1.9	3.2
Greece	28,151	0.33	8.3	61.00	67	1.3	2.06
Israel	23,578	0.386	7.3	52.2	62	4.2	
Italy	35,745	0.32	6.1	58.40	63	1.1	1.99
Malta	18,215	0.26	6.4	54.8	62	3.2	
Portugal	21,081	0.385	8.1	67.90	74	0.0	0.88
Spain	32,089	0.32	8.3	64.80	69	1.1	4.23
Turkey	9,569	0.436	8.5	n.a	55	1.9	-0.61
OECD average		0.31	7.1	66.1	66.7	1.3	0.48

Sources: GDF per capita (USD from IMF); Income inequality Human Development Report UN: Unemployment Rate (UN2007); Employment rate (European Commission, 2006); Employment rate Cyprus – Ministry of Labor, Cyprus; Employment rate Israel – Bank of Israel 2008; Total Employment, Growth Rate (UN2007); Employment rates: women (Average annual growth in percentage, 1993–2006 or latest available period) (UN2007)

Table 3 Inequality – social aspects

	CPI 2008	Female members of parliament, percent of total (2006)	Gender pay gap	Human development index (HDI)
Cyprus	5.3	14.3	n.a	0.903
Greece	4.7	13	n.a	0.926
Israel	6	14.2	36.6	0.932
Italy	4.8	17.3	n.a	0.941
Malta	5.8	9.2	6.9	0.878
Portugal	6.1	21.3	32.8	0.897
Spain	6.5	36	15.9	0.949
Turkey	4.6	4.4	n.a	0.775

Sources: CPI 2008–2008 Corruption Perceptions Index – Global Transparency: Fighting corruption for a sustainable future, High score indicates less corruption perceptions; Female members of parliament, percent of total (2006) UNECE; Gender pay gap (2006) UNECE; The Human Development Index (HDI) is an index combining normalized measures of life expectancy, literacy, educational attainment, and GDP per capita for countries worldwide

(http://www.transparency.org/policy_research/surveys_indices/cpi). The CPI data reflects the differences in corruption and in government transparency. Research (Keefer & Knack, 1996; Mauro, 1995; Brunetti, Kisunko, & Weder, 1997, pp. 23 and 25) underscores the connection between corruption and the ratio of investment per capita to GDP.

The data also refers to gender gaps in each parliament and in income. These two indicators reflect an important social cleavage. Previous research (Kaltenthaler, Ceccoli, & Gelleny, 2008; Judge & Livingston, 2008) describes gender gaps as a reflection of the degree of egalitarianism in a given society. As shown in Table 4, the Catholic countries (Italy, Portugal, and Spain) have the largest proportion of women in parliament (between 17.3 and 36%). In other countries the proportion of

Table 4 Social expenditure

	Social expenditure % GDP	Total health expenditure as % of GDP	Education spending (% of GDP)
Cyprus	18.2	6.1	6.3
Greece	24.2	9.8	4
Israel	18	7.8	7.5
Italy	26.4	8.7	4.7
Malta	18.3	8.4	n.a
Portugal	24.9	9.8	5.8
Spain	20.8	7.8	4.5
Turkey	13.2	7.7	3.7
OECD	20.9	9.0	6.2

Sources: Social expenditure % GDP Eurostat, 2005; Israel – National Insurance Institute of Israel, 2003; Turkey – www.un.org; Total health expenditure as % of GDP WHO estimates; Gross public social expenditure by broad policy area, in percentage of GDP, OECD, 2003

Scatter Plot 1 Connection between GINI coefficients for income inequality and HDI – United Nations (2009)

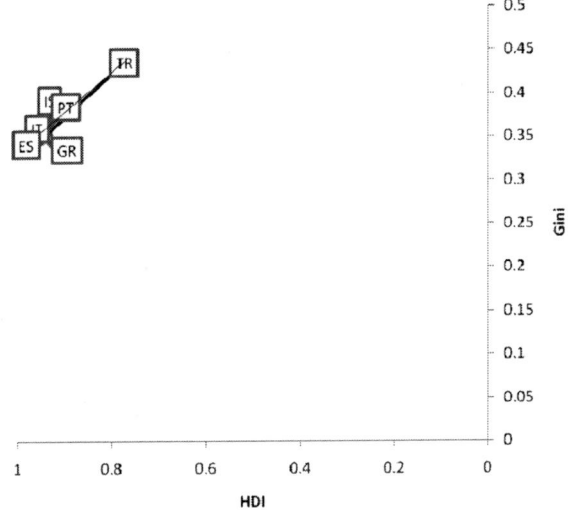

women in parliament is around 10–15%, and in Turkey, the only Muslim country, the proportion of women in parliament is very low – 4.4%. It is important to note that this indicator is also linked to gender wage discrepancies. Although data on this subject is not complete, it seems that countries with a high proportion of women in parliament have less gender wage discrepancies as compared to Turkey, for example, which has the lowest proportion of women in parliament and the highest gender wage discrepancy and income inequality.

The human development index (HDI) also indicates some differences between the eight countries: Spain, Italy, Greece, and Israel hold higher HDI rankings, while countries such as Malta and Cyprus hold slightly lower HDI rankings. It is also important to note that Turkey has the lowest HDI ranking (http://hdr.undp.org/en/media/HDR_20072008_EN_Complete.pdf). Again, a link between HDI and the GINI coefficient for income inequality can be inferred from Scatter Plot 1. HDI increases as the GINI coefficient for income inequality increases up to the GINI coefficient level of ≈0.31 (the average level of EU countries is 30.9). Above that level of GINI, the HDI begins to decrease as the GINI continues to increase. The data on Turkey, again, reflects a gloomy social condition with a GINI coefficient for income inequality of 43.9 and a poor HDI ranking.

Social Welfare in a Comparative Perspective

One of the most important indicators of the level of social welfare in a specific country is social expenditure as a percentage of GDP. This indicator reflects the state's prioritizing of social issues in terms of investment. Table 4 shows major categories of social expenditure, such as education and health, as a percentage of GDP.

The above data indicates similarities in social expenditure for seven of the eight countries (ranging from 18 to 26.4%). This data also indicates the difference between these countries and Turkey (with a social expenditure of 13.7%). It is also possible to divide the seven countries into two groups: the first group with social expenditure levels higher than 20% of total GDP (Greece, Italy, Portugal, and Spain); and the second group, with social expenditure around 18% of the total GDP (Cyprus, Israel, and Malta).

In terms of health expenditure, all the countries examined here fall within the same range – between 7.7 and 9.8% of total GDP (not including Greece with 6.1% of total GDP). On the other hand, education expenditure varies: Israel spends the largest percentage of its GDP on education (7.5% of total GDP) and is followed by Greece (6.3% of total GDP). The other countries spend between 3.7% (Turkey) and 5.8% (Portugal) of their total GDP on education.

An Example of the Relation Between Social Expenditure and Social Aspects: Gender and Inequality

As evident from Scatter Plot 2, there appears to be a connection between the wealth of the country (as reflected in GDP per capita) and its' social expenditure.

As shown, six of the eight countries reveal a linear relationship between GDP per capita and social expenditure. In the case of these countries, as GDP per capita increases social expenditure increases accordingly. While Portugal and Greece share the same tendency as the other six countries, their social expenditure actually exceeds that of countries with higher GDP per capita (such as Spain). As seen below, Scatter Plot 3 strengthens the argument regarding the connection between gender and social welfare policy.

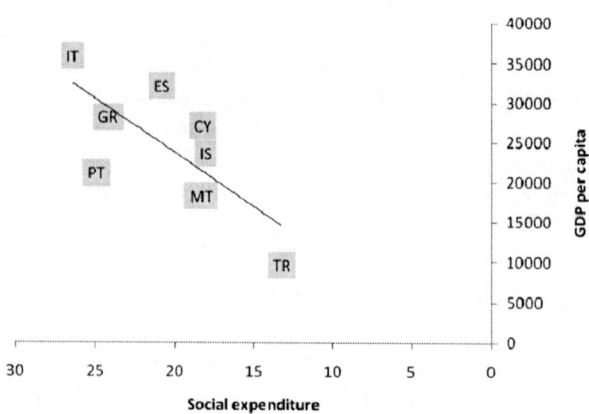

Scatter Plot 2 Connection between social expenditure and GDP per capita

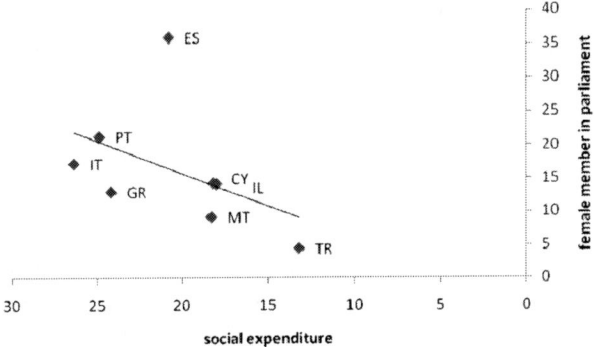

Scatter Plot 3 Connection between social expenditure and female members of parliament

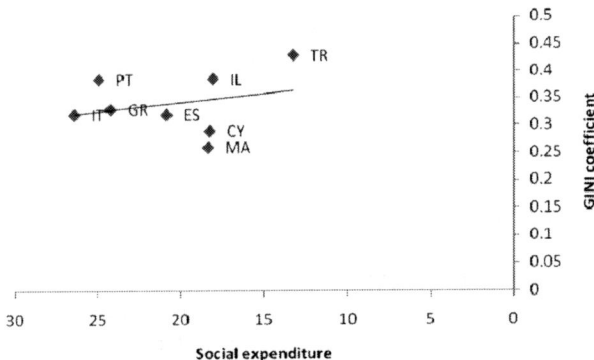

Scatter Plot 4 Connection between social expenditure and distribution of family inequality

According to this scatter plot, countries with a higher level of social expenditure also have a larger proportion of women in parliament. Nevertheless Spain and Portugal have the highest percentage of woman in parliament, but do not have the highest social expenditure rate.

One of the most interesting phenomena regarding the Mediterranean welfare state is described in Scatter Plot 4. Significant research indicates that there is a negative connection between social expenditure and social inequality. To be precise, this review indicates that a higher social expenditure rate can contribute to lower social inequality. Scatter Plot 4 generally supports this assumption, although the connection is quite small and thus weak.

Discussion: Classification of the Mediterranean Welfare States

In the attempt to classify the Mediterranean welfare states, significant conclusions emerge from the data presented in this chapter. The most obvious distinction is between Turkey, the only Muslim country in the group, and the remaining

non-Muslim countries. In almost every criterion examined in this chapter, there was
a significant difference between Turkey and the other countries. Turkey was similar
to other countries only in terms of indicators of unemployment rates and total health
expenditure as a percentage of GDP. It also bares similarity to Israel, the only other
non-Christian country, in regards to the percentage of young children.

Another way to classify these countries is by examining GDP per capita as can
be seen in Table 5.

This classification yields three groups: Group 1 includes the richest countries
(Italy and Spain), which have slightly higher levels of inequality than the EU average. HDI is high and labor force participation ranges between 63 and 69%. In
these countries social expenditure is relatively high. Group 2 includes countries of
medium wealth. This group includes four countries, Cyprus, Israel, Portugal, and
Malta. Cyprus and Malta have slightly lower inequality levels than the EU average
while Israel and Portugal have higher inequality levels than the EU average. HDI in
these countries is lower (not including Israel) as is social expenditure (not including
Portugal). Turkey is the only country in group 3, and is also the only Muslim country in this study. Turkey ranks lowest in all indicators with the exception of social
inequality, in which Turkey holds the highest rank.

This classification provides a distinction between wealthier and poorer countries
(especially countries at the extreme ends of the scale such as Turkey and Italy), but it
does not differentiate well between the wealthiest countries (such as Italy and Spain)
and countries of medium wealth (such as Israel and Portugal). It seems that there
is divergence between these countries regarding the link between GDP (wealth)
and social expenditure, and between social expenditure and inequality. While the
link between higher GDP and higher social expenditure/lower inequality holds for
the first group, the second group shows different patterns. For example, Portugal
which has a low GDP per capita has a high rate of social expenditure, but also a
high rate of inequality. Despite these differences, the connection between per capita

Table 5 Classification of countries by GDP

Country	Religion	GDP per capita	HDI	Inequality GINI coefficient	Labor force (% of total popula- tion ages 15–64)	Social expenditure % GDP
Italy	Roman Catholicism	35,745	0.941	0.32	63	26.4
Spain	Roman Catholicism	32,089	0.949	0.32	69	21.2
Greece	Greek Orthodox	28,151	0.926	0.33	67	24.2
Cyprus	Greek Orthodox	27,047	0.903	0.29	71	18.2
Israel	Jews	23,578	0.932	0.386	62	23
Portugal	Roman Catholicism	21,081	0.897	0.385	74	24.7
Malta	Roman Catholicism	18,215	0.878	0.26	62	18.3
Turkey	Muslims	9,569	0.775	0.436	55	13.7

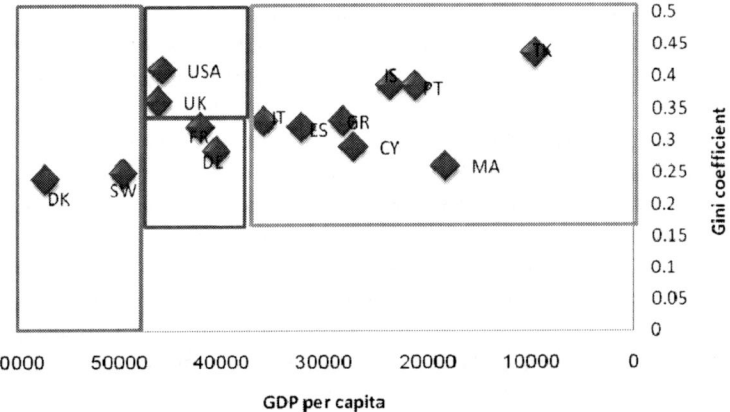

Scatter Plot 5 Connection between GDP per capita and GINI coefficient

GDP and social expenditure in the context of a comparative analysis reveals that Mediterranean welfare states differ from other European welfare states.

From Scatter Plot 5, it would appear that Mediterranean countries differ from other welfare states especially in terms of their wealth. The Mediterranean countries share similar connections between per capita GDP and social expenditure, while other welfare states do not share this connection.

Another way to distinguish between Mediterranean welfare states and other welfare states is by showing the connection between social expenditure and GDP, as described in Scatter Plot 6.

This scatter plot classifies the European welfare states into three welfare state types: the Scandinavian model, the conservative model (which, in this case, includes the UK), and the Mediterranean model. Again, it is obvious that the Mediterranean countries are not as wealthy as the other European countries. It is also clear that the

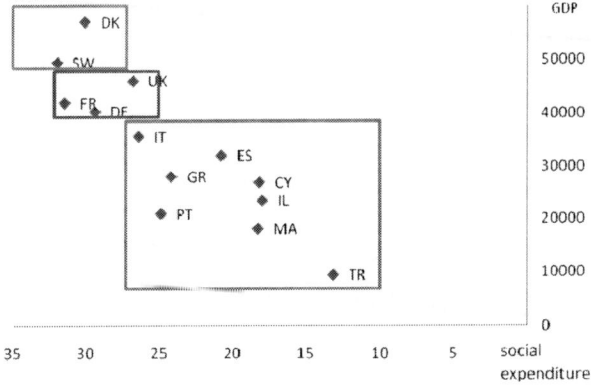

Scatter Plot 6 Connection between GDP per capita and social expenditure

social spending of these Mediterranean countries, relative to other European countries, is less. This scatter plot also corresponds with some of Esping-Andersen's (1990) assumptions regarding the extent of social expenditure and its role in distinguishing different welfare states. And finally, Scatter Plot 5 supports other findings which place Italy close to the conservative, western European welfare state type.

In conclusion, as Ferrera (1998) and Rhodes (1997) have argued, a distinct type of welfare state does in fact exist in southern Mediterranean countries. While these countries are not identical in terms of all indicators, from a comparative point of view they share an important common denominator that influences their welfare state: level of per capita GDP and social expenditure as a percentage of GDP. The fact that in the case of the southern Mediterranean welfare states these two characteristics are lower than in the "conservative" and "social democratic" welfare states indicates a welfare state category of their own.

Websites Accessed

http://w3.unece.org/pxweb/Dialog/
http://data.un.org/
http://www.who.int/research/en/
http://www.worldvaluessurvey.org/
http://www.oecd.org/statsportal/0,3352,en_2825_293564_1_1_1_1_1,00.html
http://www.imf.org/external/data.htm
http://unstats.un.org/unsd/default.htm
http://ec.europa.eu/index_en.htm
http://www.mlsi.gov.cy/mlsi/mlsi.nsf/dmlindex_en/dmlindex_en
http://www.transparency.org/policy_research/surveys_indices/cpi
http://hdr.undp.org/en/statistics/
http://www.btl.gov.il/English%20Homepage/Pages/default.aspx
http://epp.eurostat.ec.europa.eu/tgm/table.do?tab=table&language=en&
    pcode=tsiem010&tableSelection=1&footnotes=yes&labeling=labels&
    plugin=1

References

Bank of Israel. (2008). *Annual report 2007*. Jerusalem: Ayalon Printing Ltd. Retrieved from http://www.bankisrael.gov.il/deptdata/mehkar/doch07/eng/doch07e.htm

Brunetti, A., Kisunko, G., & Weder, B. (1997). *Credibility of rules and economic growth – Evidence from a world wide private sector survey*. Background paper for the World Development Report 1997. Washington, DC: The World Bank.

Esping-Andersen, G. (1990). *The three worlds of welfare capitalism*. Princeton, NJ: Princeton University Press.

Ferrera, M. (1998). The four "social Europes:" Between universalism and selectivity. In M. Rhodes & Y. Me'ny (Eds.), *The future of European welfare: A new social contract?* (pp. 79–96). New York: Palgrave.

Judge, T. A., & Livingston, B. A. (2008). Is the gap more than gender? A longitudinal analysis of gender role orientation and earning. *Journal of Applied Psychology, 93*(5), 944–1012.

Kaltenthaler, K., Ceccoli, S., & Gelleny, R. (2008). Attitudes toward eliminating income inequality in Europe. *European Union Politics, 9*(2), 217–241.

Keefer, P., & Knack, S. T. (1996). Institutions and economic performance: Cross-country tests using alternative institutional measures. *Economics and Politics, 7*, 207–227.

Lindh, T. (1999). Age structure and economic policy: The case of saving and growth. *Population Research and Policy Review, 18*(3), 261–277.

Lindh, T., & Malmberg, B. (1999). Age structure effects and growth in the OECD, 1950–1990. *Journal of Population Economics, 12*(3), 431–449.

Mauro, P. (1995). Corruption and growth. *Quarterly Journal of Economics, 110*(3), 681–712.

Rhodes, M. (1997). Southern European welfare states: Identity, problems and prospects of reform. In M. Rhodes (Ed.), *Southern European welfare state between crisis and reform* (pp. 1–22). London: Frank Cass.

United Nations. (2009). *Human Development Report 2009*. New York: Department of Social and Economic Affairs. Retrieved from http://hdrstats.undp.org/indicators/147.html

United Nations, Department of Economic and Social Affairs, Population Division. (2007). *World population prospects: The 2006 revision, highlights, working paper No. ESA/P/WP.202*. New York: United Nations. Retrieved from http://www.un.org/esa/population/publications/wpp2006/WPP2006_Highlights_rev.pdf

Name Index

Lightning Source UK Ltd.
Milton Keynes UK
18 July 2010

157167UK00003B/5/P